MFA's Standards and Guidelines for Medical Fitness Center Facilities

Medical Fitness Association

Editor
Brad Roy, PhD, FACSM, FACHE
The Summit Medical Fitness Center
Kalispell, MT

HEALTHY LEARNING

ISBN: 978-1-60679-034-2
Library of Congress Control Number: 2008941747
Cover design: Roger W. Rybkowski
Book layout: Roger W. Rybkowski
Cover photos: ©2008 Jupiter Images Corporation

Healthy Learning
P.O. Box 1828
Monterey, CA 93942
www.healthylearning.com

Contents

Editor and Editorial Board

Acknowledgments

A special thanks to the following individuals for their editorial input to this book:

William G. Herbert, Ph.D., FACSM, FAACVPR, Professor & Director, Laboratory for Health and Exercise Science, Virginia Tech, Blacksburg, VA

Thomas M. Lachocki, Ph.D., CEO, National Swimming Pool Foundation, Colorado Springs, CO

Stephen J. Tharrett, MS, Consultant, Club Industry Consulting, Dallas, TX

James A. Peterson, Ph.D., FACSM, Monterey, CA

Preface

The medical fitness industry began in the late 1970's, when several visionary hospitals recognized the need for a fitness/wellness center to serve their rapidly growing aging and physically challenged population. Since then, the medical fitness industry has grown to serve more than three million individuals in over 950 hospital affiliated centers. These facilities generally provide a higher level of medical accountability, resources, and monitoring compared to their commercial counterparts. In addition to the growing number of medical fitness centers that are directly linked to hospitals, many centers are not hospital-owned but maintain a critical and necessary affiliation with their community's healthcare delivery system. As such, given the current and future expansion of society's aging and 'health-challenged' population, the role that medical fitness centers play in reducing and preventing chronic health conditions has become increasingly critical.

The standards and guidelines presented in this document represent a set of nationally derived parameters that are applicable to the design and operation of a medical fitness facility. A number of factors can distinguish the medical fitness model from traditional health and fitness operations, including, but not limited to, active and regular medical oversight; a organizational commitment to disease management and clinical integration; and a focus on helping improve community health.

The Medical Fitness Association (MFA) was established in 1991 as a resource to the growing hospital wellness and fitness center industry, and to promote the medical fitness difference. As a nonprofit organization, the MFA assists medically integrated fitness centers in enhancing member programs and services; works to establish protocols and professional standards; acts as a resource for information and education; communicates with public and governmental bodies; renders public relations and marketing support; and encourages ethical business practices that can help improve efficiency and maximize revenue.

It is important to keep in mind that the standards and guidelines presented are intended to provide basic parameters for the prudent operation of a medical fitness center. The standards and guidelines are not intended to be a "legal" requirement, nor are they intended to present basic exercise guidelines. These are widely available in the published literature, through other professional organizations, such as the American College of Sports Medicine (ACSM), the American Association for Cardiovascular and Pulmonary Rehabilitation (AACVPR), and the American Heart Association (AHA). The standards and guidelines are neither meant to be all-inclusive nor exclusive of other operational procedures and policies that may be applicable. The MFA recognizes that special circumstances may at times necessitate deviations from the standards and guidelines presented and that the ultimate responsibility for implementing prudent policies and practices lies with each individual facility.

The standards and guidelines are designed to address two specific goals of the MFA: 1) to assist facilities in providing their participants a safe and medically sound experience that focuses on health improvement; and, 2) to develop collaborative relationships with other professional bodies (such as ACSM, ACE, and AACVPR) in order to work together to develop parameters that are complementary and consistent with each other. To this extent, the reader is encouraged to review documents published by these organizations in order to identify those policies and procedures that are most appropriate to their community and the needs of the individuals that their facility serves.

Notice and Disclaimer

The Medical Fitness Association (MFA) has developed this book to help integrated medical fitness centers to be better prepared to fulfill their unique and special mission. The standards and guidelines presented in this book are designed to serve primarily as an educational resource to assist medical fitness centers in their efforts to provide quality services and programs. Adherence to these standards and guidelines does not necessarily ensure a successful medical fitness center or client outcome. These standards and guidelines should not be considered inclusive of all proper policies, procedures and/or protocols and should not be a substitute for the medical fitness practitioner's own professional judgment to a specific client, clinical, or institutional circumstance.

The MFA and each of its past or present officers, directors, agents, servants, employees, representatives, attorneys, advisors, predecessors, successors, and assigns (hereinafter referred to individually or collectively as MFA/related parties) do not warrant or represent that the standards and guidelines, or the protocols, procedures, and information set forth in this book will, in fact, result in meeting all essential elements for facility operations, program design, or development that satisfy a minimally acceptable and otherwise safe or successful standard.

To the maximum extent permitted by applicable law, the MFA/related parties disclaim all other representations, warranties, conditions or other terms, either express or implied, including, but not limited to, implied warranties and/or conditions of merchantability and fitness for a particular purpose with regard to the use and application of the information set forth in this book or in any other regard whatsoever.

The MFA standards and guidelines or other materials and information are provided "as is" without warranty of any kind, either expressed or implied, including, but not limited to, the implied warranties of merchantability and appropriateness for a particular purpose.

The MFA/related parties shall not be liable for any direct, indirect, special, consequential, punitive, exemplary and/or incidental damages of any kind whatsoever (including, but not limited to, lost profits or attorneys' fees) resulting from the reliance on or use or other application of the standards and guidelines or other materials and information detailed in this book, even if the MFA/related parties has been advised of the possibility of such damages. This limitation applies to all causes of action in the aggregate, including, but not limited to, breach of contract, breach of warranty, negligence, strict liability, misrepresentation, and any other tort (including, without limitation, damages for personal injury, wrongful death, loss of companionship or affection, loss of a normal life, pain or suffering, disability, disfigurement, lost wages, income, profits, or any other pecuniary loss, including consequential or incidental damages).

Governing Law

This Agreement, and the respective rights and obligations of the parties hereto, shall be governed by and construed in accordance with the laws of the State of Illinois (excluding any conflict of laws provisions of the State of Illinois that would refer to and apply the substantive laws of another jurisdiction). Any suit or proceeding regarding the MFA/related parties shall be brought only in Cook County, Illinois. All parties relying on these standards and guidelines, in any respect, consent to the exclusive personal jurisdiction and venue of the court, state and federal, located in Chicago, Cook County, Illinois.

Chapter One
Integrated for Excellence

In its own way, every field of endeavor has its own unique set of circumstances. The major forces at work are distinct, the essential activities are interrelated, and the key players define the industry. The field of medical fitness is no exception.

The Growing Healthcare Crisis

Considerable evidence exists suggesting that the United States is in the midst of an ever-expanding healthcare crisis. The incidence of individuals with one or more chronic diseases is higher than it's ever been, and is growing at an alarming rate. Over one-fourth of the population suffers from cardiovascular disease. An even greater number of Americans are affected by arthritis and chronic pain and their related disability. The prevalence of obesity among both adults and children exceeds even the most pessimistic forecasts. In turn, healthcare spending is out of control, as Americans are forced to deal with the financial ramifications of the health crisis.

The Medical Fitness Association Difference

Fortunately, a viable opportunity exists to reverse the healthcare crisis in America. The essence of this approach is to place the focus and emphasis on preventing, rather than treating, disease and illness. The conceptual foundation of this approach—"exercise is medicine"—is supported and reinforced by numerous studies that show that engaging in physical activity on a regular basis provides a host of health-related benefits to individuals of all ages, fitness levels, and interests.

In response to the challenges inherent in dealing with the healthcare crisis in the United States, as well as the inexplicable fact that most Americans lead a sedentary lifestyle, the Medical Fitness Association (MFA) has developed a strategic plan that involves utilizing health and fitness programs to help prevent and manage chronic and lifestyle-related health conditions. The core of this plan entails using more than just exercise programming. Rather, the MFA's strategic approach involves providing medical oversight to the efforts to offer sound health-related programs and services. These efforts also integrate the knowledge and experience of professionals in a variety of other areas of expertise, including nutrition, mental health, physical therapy, nursing, and condition-specific medicine.

The end result of MFA's strategic thinking has been the establishment of almost 1,000 medical fitness centers across the United States. Each of these centers serves a variety of populations, offering programming and services for all ages and stages of life. Each provides rehab and post-rehab programs, as well as offerings for special populations, in addition to "traditional" exercise programming. Each focuses on the whole person, utilizing an array of strategies to reduce the risk of illness, prevent disease, and maximize health and quality of life.

The Roadmap to Excellence

MFA's Standards and Guidelines for Medical Fitness Center Facilities is designed to reinforce MFA's resolute commitment to have a positive impact on the health and quality of life of everyone it serves. The information detailed in this landmark text provides a series of "benchmarks for excellence" to help ensure that every MFA-affiliated facility is fulfilling not only its own unique mission, but also its rightful role by responsibly helping to address America's healthcare crisis.

Chapter Two
Medical Oversight

Medical oversight involves a process designed to help ensure that the programs and services provided by the medical fitness center are both safe and effective. The individual and/or group of professionals assigned responsibility for medical oversight must make certain that whoever is involved with developing the center's programming is able to integrate knowledge of the special needs of each user of a facility with appropriate assessment procedures and exercise techniques. Subsequently, all programs and services that are offered must effectively meet those needs without exposing participants to unnecessary risks.

STANDARDS AND GUIDELINES FOR MEDICAL OVERSIGHT—#1

Standard 1: *A Medical Fitness Center must have medical oversight. A medical director, a physician advisory committee, and/or a physician advisor must be in place to provide medical oversight for the facility's programming in order to maximize the safety of all participants and ensure medically and scientifically sound programs and services.*

Guidelines:

1. The facility leadership and the medical director/advisory committee should meet a minimum of four times per year.
2. The medical director/advisory committee should provide oversight for, but not restricted to:
   - Emergency-response/code policy/procedure review.
   - The AED program of the facility.
   - Staff emergency-response training.
   - Periodic review of emergency/code response outcomes and identification of opportunities for improvement.
   - Periodic review of clinical programs, policies, and clinical outcomes.
   - Periodic review of all screening programs, associated outcomes, and appropriateness of follow-up.

- Review of the facility's continuum-of-care processes with regard to the appropriateness of referrals, communication, and necessary follow-up.
- Assist in the development of clinical program content, appropriate programming and safety considerations for special populations.

STANDARDS AND GUIDELINES FOR MEDICAL OVERSIGHT —#2

Standard 2: *The clinical programs/services offered within a Medical Fitness Center must comply with the current requirements by the Centers for Medicare and Medicaid Services, such as cardiac rehabilitation phase II, physical and occupational therapy, speech therapy, and other billed clinical services including, but not limited to the requirements for physician referral, supervision, communication, documentation/charting; and patient safety.*

Guidelines:

1. The requirements of the Centers for Medicare and Medicaid services should be reviewed periodically.
2. The results of the review should be recorded and evaluated to determine whether a need for subsequent action exists.

STANDARDS AND GUIDELINES FOR MEDICAL OVERSIGHT —#3

Standard 3: *A Medical Fitness Center must demonstrate a direct and valid relationship with its community healthcare system/local continuum of care.*

Guidelines:

1. The mission statement of the center should include a commitment by the facility to participate in the local continuum of care and individual/community health improvement.
2. The facility should maintain documentation that demonstrates active participation in the local continuum of care for a minimum of one year. Documentation could include, but not be limited to:
   - Demonstration of ownership by a hospital, health system and/or physician/ physician group.
   - Referral patterns from and to physician and physician extenders for clinical services provided by the facility.
3. In addition, the facility should maintain records of:
   - Hosted community and professional education programs/seminars covering a variety of health-related topics.
   - Health-related screenings and associated results and follow-up for individuals with results outside of the normal and/or expected range.

Chapter Three
Pre-Activity Screening

Pre-activity screening involves gathering pertinent information concerning whether individuals have an increased risk of experiencing an exercise-related cardiovascular incident while engaged in physical activity. Such information can be extremely useful to medical fitness centers in at least two ways. First, it can identify those individuals who are at risk and should be referred for medical clearance before they're permitted to participate in the program offerings of the facility. Second, it can help provide a basis for discerning the most appropriate exercise prescription for a particular person.

STANDARDS AND GUIDELINES FOR PRE-ACTIVITY SCREENING—#1

Standard 1: *A Medical Fitness Center must offer each member an appropriate pre-activity screening process and refer moderate to high-risk individuals to their respective physician for medical clearance prior to participation.*

Guidelines:

1. The facility should have a systematic process of screening for chronic diseases, associated risk stratification, and the participant's potential for exercise-related injury.
2. All pre-activity screening procedures should be straightforward, easy-to-understand, and conducted in a time-efficient manner. Every feasible step should be undertaken to encourage all users to engage in the pre-screening process.
3. All facility users should be offered a pre-activity screening prior to their participation in physical activities at the center. If a user should decline the pre-activity screening, that person should be permitted to sign a waiver for the screening that allows that individual to participate in the program offerings of the center.
4. The waiver for individuals who refuse to participate in the pre-activity screening should clearly delineate that the person has been offered a pre-activity screening; has been informed of the basic risks involved in

participating; has chosen not to follow the guidance provided by the center's staff; has assumed responsibility for his/her own actions; and has released the center from any legal responsibility from claims or suits arising from his/her participation in the center's programs.

STANDARDS AND GUIDELINES FOR PRE-ACTIVITY SCREENING—#2

Standard 2: *If the pre-activity screening identifies a potential user as having a known cardiovascular, metabolic or pulmonary disease and/or is identified as a high-risk individual, the user should be advised, in writing, to consult with a physician and/or qualified healthcare provider, and provide documentation of such consult to the facility prior to participating in physical activity at the facility.*

Guidelines:

1. All facility users who are identified as having risk factors that necessitate referral for medical consultation who fail to obtain such consultation should be permitted to sign a waiver that allows them to participate in the program offerings of the facility.
2. To the extent permitted by law, such users who refuse to sign the waiver should be precluded from participating in the program activities of the facility.

STANDARDS AND GUIDELINES FOR PRE-ACTIVITY SCREENING—#3

Standard 3: *The pre-activity screen should be reviewed and interpreted by qualified staff and the results documented, including referral to a qualified healthcare provider and the outcome of such consultation.*

Guidelines:

1. The results of the pre-activity screening should be utilized to identify and make appropriate decisions about what constitutes safe activity levels and modalities for that particular person.
2. Consistent with the Health Insurance Portability and Accountability Act of 1996 (HIPPA), a form that details a user's health information and offers a means for explicitly recording medical clearance (if given by an appropriate medical professional) should be provided by the facility to the individual to take to a physician.

Chapter Four
Risk Management and Emergency-Response Policies and Procedures

Risk management refers to the practices and systems that organizations put in place to help reduce and/or eliminate their exposure to liability and financial loss. In medical fitness centers, risk management involves the policies, practices, and procedures by which a facility reduces its risk of an employee or user experiencing an event that could result in harm to the individual or the facility itself.

Emergency-response policies and practices are an integral part of a sound risk-management system. Collectively, they are designed to help ensure that a medical fitness center's ability to respond to untoward events provides the maximum reasonable level of safety for users and staff.

STANDARDS AND GUIDELINES FOR RISK MANAGEMENT & EMERGENCY-RESPONSE POLICIES AND PROCEDURES—#1

Standard 1: *The Medical Fitness Center must have a written emergency-response plan that enables a timely and appropriate response to any emergency event that threatens the health and safety of facility users.*

Guidelines:

1. The emergency-response plan should specify the most likely emergency situations that could occur and how each circumstance will be handled, including the precise responsibilities of the first, second, and third responders to a particular emergency.
2. The emergency-response plan should be fully detailed in writing and maintained in an area easily accessed by center staff. The plan should also

include procedures for documenting in writing the fact that the emergency-response system is reviewed on a regular basis by every member of the facility's staff.

3. The facility should have a prompt and direct link to the "911" emergency-response center. Staff members should be made aware of the locations for all emergency equipment, including the facility's telephones.
4. The facility should have an adequate number of first-aid kits and other necessary emergency equipment including documentation that all equipment is periodically checked for functionality.
5. The facility should hold regular emergency drills (e.g., at least four times a year) and maintain associated documentation that demonstrates the competencies of staff to respond to emergency situations.
6. The facility should have a formal incident reporting and management program in place.
7. The facility should have signs and information in place to alert facility users to the emergency-response system.
8. The emergency-response plan should be developed in concert with and coordinated with the local emergency medical services (EMS) provider in the area of the facility.

STANDARDS AND GUIDELINES FOR RISK MANAGEMENT & EMERGENCY-RESPONSE POLICIES AND PROCEDURES—#2

Standard 2: *With physician oversight in place, a Medical Fitness Center must have an appropriate number of automated external defibrillators (AEDs) that are easily accessible for use.*

Guidelines:

1. The number of AEDs and the placement of the AEDs in a facility is a determinant of the response time/distance for the AED to be brought to the victim. The American Heart Association recommends a response time of three minutes or less. As a rule of thumb, an AED should be located within a 1.5-minute walk to any place it could potentially be needed.
2. All staff should have current CPR/AED training. At least one staff member with current CPR/AED training should be on duty during all operating hours of the facility.
3. Each AED should be maintained according to the manufacturer's guidelines and maintenance and monitoring documentation kept current.
4. Review and practice sessions to ensure that all center staff possess the appropriate skills for safely using an AED should be held on a periodic basis (e.g., once every three months).

STANDARDS AND GUIDELINES FOR RISK MANAGEMENT & EMERGENCY-RESPONSE POLICIES AND PROCEDURES—#3

Standard 3: *A Medical Fitness Center with aquatics areas must have specific written emergency plans for each pool.*

Guidelines:

1. Written policies and procedures should be developed that specify the responsibilities of staff for handling emergencies in the aquatics areas of the facility including the role of first, second, and third responder.
2. Staff should be provided regular training opportunities for water-related emergencies, with associated documentation that demonstrates the competencies of staff to respond in an appropriate manner to aquatic-emergency situations.
3. A review of the emergency system for responding to emergencies in the aquatics areas of the facility should be periodically undertaken to ensure that the policies and procedures are appropriate and are fully understood by staff.
4. All aquatics staff and volunteers conducting programs and activities in the facility's aquatic areas should meet the criteria established by the YMCA (2003) for such personnel.
5. The facility should take documented steps to warn users of actions that pose potential risks to their health and safety, including head-first entry, breath-holding, and underwater swimming.
6. The facility should develop and implement specific policies that guarantee adequate supervision of children seven years old or less while they're in aquatics areas.
7. The facility should develop a policy and procedure for handling fecal-accidents in aquatics areas.
8. The facility should develop a detailed plan to minimize the risk of potential entrapments and entanglements in the aquatics areas.

Chapter Five
Programs and Services

Within a medical fitness center, programming generally ranges from formal intervention/rehabilitation programs (e.g., cardiac rehabilitation, physical therapy, occupational therapy) to developing activities that either serve as a transition between clinical interventions/rehabilitation and fitness programming (according to generally accepted prescription guidelines) and those that address prevention, health-risk reduction, and therapeutic lifestyle factors. The growing trend of individuals who join medical fitness centers (without being directed to do so by a physician) because of the innumerable benefits such facilities offer indicates that programming also involves engaging users in the center's experience and creating opportunities for members to become actively involved in the facility.

As such, programming has the ability to create connections between users, establish training partnerships, offer competitive challenges for most individuals (within themselves and against others), and entertain the users. All factors considered, programming is the facility's most viable option for meeting and exceeding the expectations that most individuals have about being a member of a medical fitness center. Furthermore, effective clinical and non-clinical programming is also one of the best strategies a facility has for differentiating itself from its competitors, for example, a "traditional" health/fitness club.

STANDARDS AND GUIDELINES FOR PROGRAMS AND SERVICES—#1

Standard 1: *A Medical Fitness Center must have programs and services that address the needs and interests of its users.*

Guidelines:

1. The facility should have programs for persons with chronic medical conditions such as heart disease (CAD, CHF), pulmonary disease, cancer, chronic pain, orthopedic and/or neurologic problems (e.g., arthritis, fibromyalgia, osteoporosis, MS), cerebrovascular disease (stroke), sports injury prevention and rehabilitation, nutritional counseling, etc.

2. All treatments/interventions for facility participants should be based on and adhere to nationally accepted guidelines.
3. Each program should have appropriate inclusion and exclusion criteria.
4. Participants should undergo a documented initial assessment with follow-up reporting to the referring physician and/or healthcare provider.
5. Programs should provide nutritional counseling by qualified staff, when appropriate.
6. Appropriate mental-health counseling should be available to clinical program participants, as necessary, either provided by the facility, through the participant's primary care physician and/or by referral to a mental-health provider.
7. The facility should offer educational workshops/classes for clinical program participants and, when appropriate, family members.
8. Staff should maintain an open line of communication with referring physicians and other medical providers to provide members with optimal care and programming. Periodic follow-up with referring healthcare providers and/or primary care providers, as appropriate, should be encouraged and documented.
9. The facility should have policies and procedures in place that protect the confidentiality of all patients/clients and comply with all HIPAA standards of privacy and confidentiality for medical information.
10. The facility should have educational workshops/classes in place for the community that utilize healthcare professionals from the community, as well as staff expertise.
11. The facility should have lifestyle modification programs that are available for members and the community at large.

STANDARDS AND GUIDELINES FOR PROGRAMS AND SERVICES—#2

Standard 2: *A Medical Fitness Center with aquatics facilities must have written policies and procedures specific to the programs and services that are to be offered in each aquatics area.*

Guidelines:

1. These policies and procedures should include, but are not limited to, basic rules/regulations for pool use; emergency procedures; and pool and program/class supervision guidelines.

Chapter Six
Professional Staffing

Medical fitness centers tend to require a diverse array of talent to deliver the results and experiences that members desire, expect, need, and deserve. As such, centers must have employees who have an appropriate blend of education, certified technical expertise and hands-on work experience. Without exception, every professional staff member must have the ability and competencies to perform the role and responsibilities assigned to them. Because the programming that facilities provide covers such a broad spectrum of experiences, a vast pool of talent with expertise in a broad range of services is often required. Among the key attributes that are required of staff members of medical fitness centers (depending upon their position) is having a certification that has been earned from an organization that is accredited by the NCCA.

Certification Accreditation

Currently, numerous "certification" opportunities exist for non-licensed health and fitness professionals. With the ever-expanding aging population and the rapid increase in the number of people with chronic disease that are referred to and utilize medical fitness facilities, it is critical that MFA's standards and guidelines for medical fitness center facilities recommend certifications for programs that have successfully completed a rigorous accreditation process.

The meticulous evaluation of the certification process is essential in assisting professionals and medical fitness consumers in differentiating between the large numbers of certification programs currently available. In that regard, the Medical Fitness Association recognizes accreditation programs that focus on the certification processes and systems that delineate professional roles, scope of practice, exam content, and administration/scoring to ensure that:

- The examination process is fair and unbiased.
- The examination accurately measures the minimal competence of the candidate for the profession.
- The public is protected from unqualified or ineffective practitioners.
- The organization has the means to support its certified professionals.

The National Commission for Certifying Agencies (NCCA), a division of the National Organization for Competency Assurance (NOCA), has been identified as an accrediting organization that provides such a rigorous evaluation process for accreditation of professional certifications. By earning an NCCA-accredited certification, health and fitness professionals demonstrate that they are qualified to participate as part of the healthcare continuum, based on what is usual and customary for other healthcare professionals.

STANDARDS AND GUIDELINES FOR PROFESSIONAL STAFFING—#1

Standard 1: *Qualifications.* *A Medical Fitness Center must employ one or more professional(s) who hold degree(s), certification(s) and/or license(s) appropriate to each program offered and the populations served.*

Guidelines:

1. Fitness directors, managers, or supervisors should hold the following minimum qualifications:
   - Education: Bachelor's degree in exercise science or related field; master's degree preferred
   - Certification: Current fitness instructor, personal trainer, or higher certification that is accredited by the NCCA
2. Fitness instructors/staff should hold the following minimum qualifications:
   - Education: College certificate or associate's degree in exercise science; bachelor's degree in exercise science or related field preferred
   - Certification: Fitness instructor, personal trainer certification, or its equivalent that is accredited by the NCCA
3. Personal training staff should hold the following minimum qualifications:
   - Education: College certificate or associate's degree; bachelor's degree in exercise science or related field preferred
   - Certification: Fitness instructor, personal trainer certification, or its equivalent that is accredited by the NCCA
4. Clinical fitness staff providing programming for special populations should hold the following additional qualifications:
   - Cardiopulmonary rehabilitation, and/or other chronic disease program:
     - ✓ Education: Bachelor's degree in exercise science or related field; master's degree preferred
     - ✓ Certification/licensure: Professional NCCA-accredited clinical certification and/or licensed RN or PT with exercise science background; or, for pulmonary rehabilitation, licensed RT
     - ✓ Experience/training: Additional training and/or credential specific to the target population

- Orthopedic rehabilitation/post rehabilitation:
  - ✓ Education: Bachelor's degree in exercise science, physical therapy, or athletic training; master's degree preferred
  - ✓ Certification/Licensure: Professional clinical certification that is NCCA accredited and/or licensed RN, PT assistant, PT, or ATC
- Weight loss:
  - ✓ Education: Bachelor's degree in nutrition; additional course work or degree in exercise science preferred
  - ✓ Certification/licensure: RD license preferred; NCCA-accredited certification (e.g., fitness instructor or personal trainer) and specialty certificate in nutrition/weight loss
  - ✓ Staff must maintain compliance with the applicable specific State Practice Act.

5. Group-exercise instructors should hold the following minimum qualifications:
   - Education: College certificate or associate's degree in fitness/exercise science; bachelor's degree in exercise science or related field preferred
   - Certification: Group-exercise instructor or leader certification that is NCCA accredited
   - Certificate of completion or specialty certificates from a reputable organization for each specialized group modality that the instructor teaches (e.g., spinning/group cycling)
6. The aquatics director/supervisor should hold the following minimum qualifications:
   - Education: College certificate or associate's degree in fitness/exercise science; bachelor's degree in exercise science, recreation, or related field preferred
   - Certification: Current YMCA, Red Cross, or other nationally recognized certification; certification as an aquatics facility operator; certification as a pool operator, advanced life-saving certification, and/or water safety instructor certification
7. Aquatics staff should hold the following minimum qualifications:
   - Certification: Appropriate aquatics certification or specialty training certificate for position/responsibilities (e.g., lifeguard, swim instructor, WSI, aquatics exercise instructor)

STANDARDS AND GUIDELINES FOR PROFESSIONAL STAFFING—#2

Standard 2: *All staff must maintain a current certificate in automated external defibrillation (AED) and cardiopulmonary resuscitation (CPR) from a qualified certifying organization.*

Guidelines:

1. A facility should provide a specific opportunity (i.e., expenses reimbursed, release time, etc.) for each staff member to obtain an AED/CPR certificate.

2. A procedure to ensure that every staff member's AED/CPR certificate is current should be implemented.
3. Facilities should provide professional liability insurance for staff and/or encourage staff to maintain individual policies.

STANDARDS AND GUIDELINES FOR PROFESSIONAL STAFFING—#3

Standard 3: *Staff Training/Continuing Education.* *A Medical Fitness Center must provide a variety of training/continuing education opportunities for staff, utilizing relationships with and expertise of, physicians, other community healthcare professionals and/or experts, conferences, and distance learning programs that are approved for CECs.*

Guidelines:

1. A facility should provide one or more of the following for each professional staff member:
   - Periodic travel/educational opportunities for staff to attend conferences, observe seminars, make site visits, etc.
   - Facility-sponsored workshops, seminars, conferences for staff and other health professionals
   - Current literature resources/medical library access
   - Web-based/online training opportunities

STANDARDS AND GUIDELINES FOR PROFESSIONAL STAFFING—#4

Standard 4: *A Medical Fitness Center must demonstrate that all staff maintain current certification(s)/license(s) by meeting the continuing education requirements for their specific certifying/licensing bodies.*

Guidelines:

1. All certified and/or licensed professional fitness staff should maintain the following:
   - Current NCCA-accredited certification/license
   - Current CPR/AED card
   - Annual Universal Precautions training
2. The facility should have a process in place to ensure that all staff credentials are current.

Chapter Seven
Operational Policies and Practices

Operational policies and practices involve those administrative steps, procedures, and systems that enable and empower employees to deliver the medical fitness center's products and services to its users as consistently and prudently as possible. Operating practices range from the policies governing the scheduling of appointments to the practice of conducting new user orientations. The more formalized these operating practices are, the easier it is for the facility to consistently deliver its products and services. In reality, no one best method for operating a facility exists. Instead, there are benchmarks or best practices that can help clearly define what center operators should do in order to run their business successfully. The most successful facility operators typically divide operations into two basic components: base parameters and systems. The operating base parameters are the minimum expectations that a facility has for the delivery of a practice. These expectations provide a basic action framework for the staff. The systems are the tools that the staff can employ to meet the established parameters or expectations.

STANDARDS AND GUIDELINES FOR OPERATIONAL POLICIES AND PRACTICES—#1

Standard 1: *A Medical Fitness Center must have a system in place that accurately monitors who has entered and remains in the facility at any given time.*

Guidelines:

1. A procedure should be implemented to ensure that every individual in the facility has appropriate access privileges.
2. All guests and visitors should be required to check-in.
3. All non-authorized users should be required to either complete a pre-activity screening instrument or sign a waiver.
4. The number of staff scheduled to be present in the facility should be adjusted, as appropriate, in response to usage rate data.

STANDARDS AND GUIDELINES FOR OPERATIONAL POLICIES AND PRACTICES—#2

Standard 2: *A Medical Fitness Center must have a system in place for helping ensure that every user achieves the maximum benefits of their exercise and program participation efforts.*

Guidelines:

1. The facility should employ accepted methods to assess functional capacity, body, composition, muscular fitness, flexibility, balance, and other components of physical and motor fitness:
   - The facility should offer exercise testing for fitness assessments, as well as for exercise prescription purposes.
   - All fitness testing should be conducted and interpreted by qualified staff, according to industry accepted methods/protocols.
2. The facility should use the results of a user's fitness testing as a starting point for developing an appropriate exercise prescription for that individual and as a basis for monitoring progress in the program.
3. All facility users should be offered an initial orientation to the facility, facility equipment, basic program concepts, and emergency/safety guidelines.

STANDARDS AND GUIDELINES FOR OPERATIONAL POLICIES AND PRACTICES—#3

Standard 3: *A Medical Fitness Center must comply with all local, state, and federal laws and regulations governing the operation of their facility including—but not limited to—building codes, ADA, OHSA, etc.*

Guidelines:

1. A facility should have an appropriate level of air circulation and air quality.
2. A facility should have an appropriate level of illumination to help ensure that a reasonably safe environment for engaging in physical activity exists.
3. A facility should have a reasonable amount of access space between equipment and activity areas.
4. A facility should separate activity areas from spaces devoted to maintenance, storage, and front-of-the-house and back-of-the-house operations.
5. A facility should have an appropriate number of restrooms.
6. A facility should have wall and floor surfaces in its activity areas that minimize the risk of injury to participants.
7. The facility should be accessible to the disabled.

8. Facility equipment should be inclusive to allow the majority of the disabled access to a full-body workout.
9. Staff should be provided training to augment their understanding of the needs of the disabled and various age groups such as children and the elderly.
10. Facility should annually conduct an accessibility survey utilizing disabled persons and document efforts to enhance facility accessibility.
11. A facility should conduct preventative maintenance on all of its exercise equipment according to guidelines provided by the equipment's manufacturer. A written record of the maintenance inspection and follow-up should be kept for at least a year. All safety concerns involving equipment in the facility should be appropriately addressed in a timely manner.

STANDARDS AND GUIDELINES FOR OPERATIONAL POLICIES AND PRACTICES—#4

Standard 4: *A Medical Fitness Center with aquatics facilities must comply with all local and state laws/regulations regarding pool chemistry, chemical storage, pool supervision, signage, etc.*

Guidelines:

1. Facilities should employ or contract with at least one staff person who is a certified pool operator (CPO).
2. Pool chemistry should be checked on a regular basis, as required by state/local regulations, and documentation should be maintained and recorded.
3. Signage should be posted in easily viewed areas and include pool user rules/regulations, appropriate warnings and emergency procedures.
4. Facilities should maintain and follow a written fecal accident policy and educate users regarding the importance of following pool hygiene rules.
5. Chemicals should be stored in appropriately secured locations and in a manner consistent with state laws and regulations.
6. Material safety data sheet(s) (MSDS) should be posted and/or available in the aquatics chemical storage area, and be readily obtainable by all staff members.

STANDARDS AND GUIDELINES FOR OPERATIONAL POLICIES AND PRACTICES—#5

Standard 5: *A Medical Fitness Center must meet all current local code, state and OSHA requirements for potentially hazardous materials, including handling of bodily fluids.*

Guidelines:

1. Material safety data sheets, for each potentially hazardous material should be maintained and readily available to all staff members. Staff should receive regular training/review in handling potentially hazardous materials, at least on an annual basis.
2. The facility should provide and document staff training regarding the appropriate handling of bodily fluids and cleaning of contaminated surfaces.
3. A facility should conduct and document a safety audit at regular intervals and review the results with the medical director or medical advisory committee.

Chapter Eight
Signage

Medical fitness centers can reduce their level of business risk and, at the same time, help create a safer physical activity environment for their users by developing signage that is then posted in appropriate locations that communicates to its users those areas of the facility that involve a potentially substantial risk to an individual's health and safety. This signage should indicate the risks involved and include information that can lessen the individual's risk if they respond appropriately to the information provided to them. Detailed information on developing proper signage for the exercise-related facilities has been developed by and is available from the American Society for Testing and Materials.

STANDARDS AND GUIDELINES FOR SIGNAGE—#1

Standard 1: *A Medical Fitness Center must conspicuously post the appropriate signage indicating caution, danger, and warning in those locations that warrant such signage.*

Guidelines:

1. A facility should post signage (in every activity area in which such signage is appropriate) that alerts users that a specific activity may expose them to an increased level of risk. Examples of signage commonly included in key areas of a facility include the following:
   - Sauna, steam room, and whirlpool:
     - ✓ Information about the temperature range to which the user will be exposed
     - ✓ A warning about the increased risk of hyperthermia if too much time is spent in any of these facilities
     - ✓ A warning about specific populations who should avoid exposure to these areas unless they have their physician's approval, such as those individuals with either high blood pressure or coronary artery disease, women who are pregnant, members on vasodilating medications, etc.
     - ✓ A warning to cool down after exercise before entering these areas
     - ✓ Guidelines on what constitutes a reasonably safe time period for individuals to utilize these areas

- Aquatics areas:
  - ✓ A warning about not running or playing on the pool deck
  - ✓ A warning about deck surfaces being slippery when wet
  - ✓ A warning about no diving
  - ✓ Information about food not being allowed around the pool
  - ✓ Information that no supervision or lifeguard is present (if the pool is not required by law to have lifeguards)
  - ✓ Information about not entering the pool immediately after eating
  - ✓ Information about showering before entering the pool

With regard to signage for aquatics areas, facility operators should be familiar with the local laws and regulations to ensure that their facilities are in full compliance with all the legally required signage expectations.

- Enclosed racquet courts (e.g., handball, racquetball, and squash):
  - ✓ Signage that indicates that individuals should wear appropriate eye protection when using the courts
- Fitness areas:
  - ✓ Recommendation to have a spotter when performing certain free-weight exercises (free-weight area)
  - ✓ Recommendation to get instruction or guidance from a professional before embarking on a fitness program
  - ✓ Recommendation to stop exercising if the individual experiences dizziness, pain, or unusual discomfort
  - ✓ Instructional signage that helps enhance the safety level of a particular piece of equipment
  - ✓ Signage that indicates when a piece of equipment is out of order

In addition to signage in the fitness areas that focuses on the aforementioned information and warnings, facilities should also provide either perceived-exertion charts or target heart-rate charts so that users can monitor their level of exertion while exercising.

- Hazardous conditions signage:
  - ✓ When equipment is out of order and the facility wants to make sure its members are aware that the equipment is out of service
  - ✓ When floors are wet and the facility wants to make its members/users aware of slippery conditions
  - ✓ When a condition exists, such as damaged walking surfaces, loose impediment, or a related condition that would increase the risk to the facility's users
  - ✓ When repairs or construction are being performed and the facility wants to warn its members/users of specific dangers and/or locations to avoid

2. All such signage should have the required signal icon, signal word, signal color, and layout, as specific by the American National Standards Institute (ANSI).

STANDARDS AND GUIDELINES FOR SIGNAGE—#2

Standard 2: *A Medical Fitness Center must post all required ADA and OSHA signage.*

Guidelines:

1. A facility should provide signage that indicates access points for individuals with physical challenges.
2. A facility should provide signage that can be viewed by those individuals who have impaired vision.
3. A facility should provide signage that informs individuals of the possible exposure to hazardous chemicals and blood-borne chemicals.

STANDARDS AND GUIDELINES FOR SIGNAGE—#3

Standard 3: *A Medical Fitness Center must post signage involving fire and related emergency situations, as required by local, state, and federal regulations and codes.*

Guidelines:

1. A facility should post signage indicating certificate of occupancy.
2. A facility should post emergency exit signage.
3. A facility should post signage indicating the location of emergency phone(s), fire extinguisher(s), AED units, and first-aid equipment.
4. A facility should work closely with their local fire department and city officials to ensure that it is in complete compliance with the requirement for fire and emergency situation signage.

Chapter Nine
Quality Management

Quality management involves developing and adhering to a set of policies and procedures that are designed to help determine whether a particular program, service, or a measure of organizational performance or outcome is meeting a defined set of expectations and/or requirements. Quality management is used by medical fitness centers to help ensure that their program offerings and organizational undertakings are of the highest quality.

STANDARDS AND GUIDELINES FOR QUALITY MANAGEMENT—#1

Standard 1: *A Medical Fitness Center must have a systematic process in place to continuously assess and improve all aspects of health and fitness delivery, including, but not limited to, individual user outcomes, clinical and non-clinical programs/services, and operational/business processes.*

Guidelines:

1. Quality management: The facility should have a policy and procedure in place for ensuring that all activities involving a particular program/service/process are effective and efficient with respect to expectations and the facility's mission, stated goals, and objectives.
2. A facility's quality management program should provide coordination, integration, and support for performance improvement activities throughout the center and ensure participation by all departments and services in order to help accomplish the following:
   - Achieve a collaborative process in the design of new services, programs, or processes.
   - Identify and utilize key findings to improve performance, key processes, and member/patient/user experience and safety.
   - Minimize delays, errors, and rework in providing services by focusing improvement efforts on the well-planned, cost-effective, and service-oriented progression of each individual through the health and fitness experience.

- Assure communication and reporting among facility administration, physicians and other healthcare providers, managers/supervisors, staff, and medical director/advisory committees.
- Provide for rapid identification and prevention of adverse user experiences, and facilitate optimal management through coordination of appropriate responses.
- Identify and address user/patient, partner, and community needs in accordance with the facility's mission.

3. A facility's quality management program should provide for regular reporting, oversight, and publishing of performance improvement activities and associated results, such as:
   - General program and individual member results and outcomes
   - Compliance with stated goals with major reasons for successes and failures
   - Reason(s) for the termination of program(s)
   - Member and program participant survey data and identified opportunities for improvement
   - Key implemented projects designed to improve performance
4. Performance improvement: The facility should have a standardized method of measuring and evaluating the output/outcome of programs, procedures, and processes and for modifying each, based on the results, to increase its effectiveness and performance. Facility goals and objectives and state, regional, and/or national data, if available, should be used as benchmarks during the process.
5. Performance improvement/outcome data should be measured, evaluated, acted upon, and documented in the following, but not limited to the following areas:
   - Safety/emergency-response/sentinel events
   - Individual member/user outcomes:
     - ✓ Referrals to and from physicians and healthcare providers
     - ✓ Pre-activity screenings
     - ✓ Expanded health-risk appraisals
     - ✓ Fitness testing/evaluations (blood pressure, blood glucose, weight/BMI/body composition, lipids, exercise tests, etc.)
     - ✓ Exercise and other risk-factor/lifestyle-change programming
   - Facility programs:
     - ✓ Clinical and non-clinical programs/services
     - ✓ Health-related seminars/classes/programs
     - ✓ Health-related screenings (BP, glucose, cholesterol, prostate cancer, skin cancer, etc.)

- Surveys:
  - ✓ Member satisfaction
  - ✓ Patient-satisfaction measures
  - ✓ Seminar/class/program
  - ✓ Employee satisfaction
- Business processes and performance
- Benchmarks/standards of performance for organizational operations, such as:
  - ✓ Operating margin
  - ✓ Labor as a percent of revenue
  - ✓ Volumes
  - ✓ FTEs
  - ✓ FTE and or salary per unit (visit, etc.)
  - ✓ Expense per unit (visit, etc.)
  - ✓ Supplies per unit
  - ✓ Revenue per unit
  - ✓ Revenue per square foot
  - ✓ EBITDA
- Annual budget and associated performance
- Goals/objectives and key strategies
- Human resource-related factors, such as:
  - ✓ Turnover rates
  - ✓ Productivity
  - ✓ Absenteeism
  - ✓ Employee satisfaction

Appendix A
Supplements

A-1. Sample Medical Oversight Committee Structure

A-2. Sample Medical Emergency Policies and Procedures
- Code Blue
- Code Yellow
- Code Red
- Code Strong
- Code Black
- Code Purple

A-3. AED & CPR Training Plan

A-4. Sample Safety-Inspection Program

A-5. Sample Job Descriptions
- Facility Director/General Manager
- Medical Director
- Fitness Manager/Director/Supervisor
- Fitness Instructor
- Personal Trainer
- Aquatics Director
- Aquatics Staff (Lifeguard)
- Group-Exercise Coordinator/Director
- Group-Fitness Instructor
- Front-Desk Receptionist
- Supervisor on Duty (SOD)

A-6. Sample Centers for Medicare and Medicaid Services Guideline

A-7. 101 Reasons to Exercise

Appendix A-1
Sample Medical Oversight Committee Structure

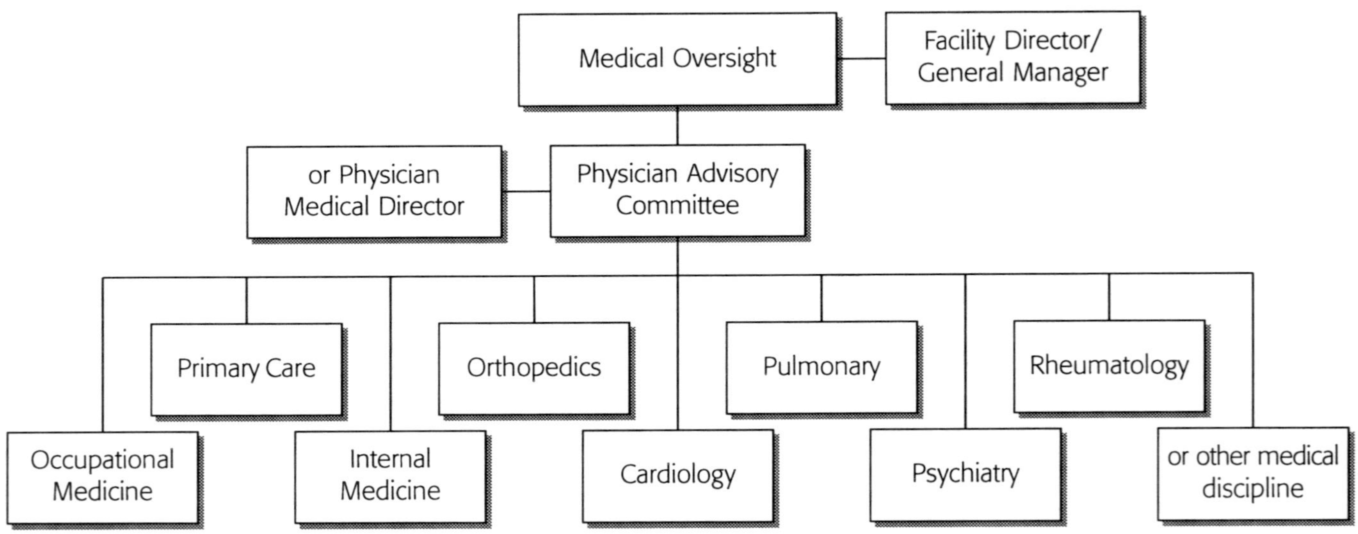

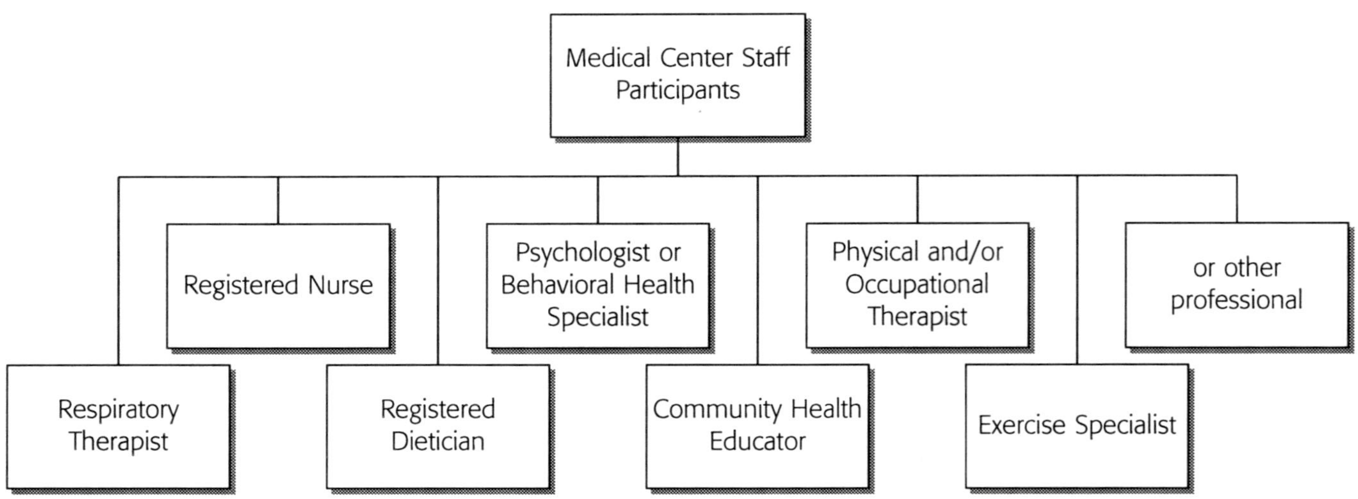

Appendix A-2
Sample Medical Emergency Policies and Procedures

A-2a. Code Blue (Unresponsive Victim)

(Facility Name)

POLICY AND PROCEDURE:

MANUAL: *(Facility Name)* Policy & Procedures Manual *(Facility Name)* Safety Manual	**POLICY NO.:** ____	
EFFECTIVE:	**SUBJECT:** Code Blue (Unresponsive Victim)	
REVIEWED:	**DIVISION:** *(Facility Name)*	
REVISED:	**ISSUING DEPT.:**	**DISTRIBUTION:** All ________ Departments
APPROVED DIRECTOR: **DATE:**	**APPROVED DEPT. MANAGER:** **DATE:**	

PURPOSE:

1. To respond appropriately to unresponsive victims
2. To identify the skills and roles pertinent to a resuscitative response
3. To provide for documentation of resuscitation events
4. To promote continuous improvement in resuscitation services

POLICY:

1. All *(Facility Name)* staff will be familiar with Basic Life Support procedures and shall be currently trained in Heartsaver AED or higher level. All staff not trained in the use of the AED shall receive such training at the time of the next renewal period.
2. Any staff person who observes an individual in cardiac arrest shall initiate Code Blue procedure as described below.
3. Code Blue events shall be documented per *(Facility Name)* incident reporting policy, and shall be reviewed as soon after the event as possible with all involved parties.

PROCEDURE:

1. Confirm unresponsiveness of the victim.
2. Initiate Code Blue protocol:
   A. Call or have someone else call 9-9-1-1.
   B. Send someone to the front desk to report Code Blue.
   C. Send someone to retrieve the oxygen and the AED from *(specific location)*.
   D. Use universal precautions/body substance isolation technique and begin resuscitation.
   E. Begin AED protocol upon arrival of the AED at the scene.
   F. Continue resuscitation efforts until relieved by EMS personnel.
3. Upon receiving a report of Code Blue, the front desk will page "Code Blue to location" three times, using the overhead emergency paging system.
4. The on-call supervisor (MOD) will take charge of the scene and direct the actions of responders.
5. The Patient Care Action Log will be maintained until the patient is transported by EMS personnel.
6. AED and BLS supplies used in the resuscitation will be checked and restocked as necessary by on-call supervisor
7. The patient care action log will be delivered to *(Facility Name)* administration for director/manager review

PERFORMANCE IMPROVEMENT:

1. Code events will be evaluated by the response team and the *(Facility Name)* manager/director.
2. The entire process will be evaluated for timeliness, appropriateness, efficiency, and outcome.
3. Deficiencies will be noted, and methods for improvement implemented.
4. All code events will be reported to and reviewed by the physician advisory committee.

A-2b. Code Yellow (Medical Emergency, Non-Code Blue)

(Facility Name)

POLICY AND PROCEDURE:

<table>
<tr><td>MANUAL: (Facility Name) Safety Manual

(Facility Name) Policy & Procedures Manual</td><td colspan="2">POLICY NO.: ____</td></tr>
<tr><td>EFFECTIVE:</td><td colspan="2">SUBJECT: Code Yellow (Medical Emergency, Non-Code Blue)</td></tr>
<tr><td>REVIEWED:</td><td colspan="2">DIVISION: (Facility Name)</td></tr>
<tr><td>REVISED:</td><td>ISSUING DEPT.:</td><td>DISTRIBUTION:

All _________ Departments</td></tr>
<tr><td>APPROVED DIRECTOR:

DATE:</td><td colspan="2">APPROVED DEPT. MANAGER:

DATE:</td></tr>
</table>

PURPOSE:

To insure that all patrons and/or staff who become injured or suddenly ill are given appropriate medical attention or are instructed how/where/when to receive such care prior to leaving ______________________ *(Facility Name)* property

POLICY:

1. All *(Facility Name)* staff shall be familiar with basic life support and Code Yellow procedures.
2. All *(Facility Name)* staff shall assist patrons or other staff members who become injured or ill to the extent of their level of training as necessary.
3. *(Facility Name)* staff shall initiate "Code Yellow" response when indicated and will not attempt to care for injured/ill persons single-handedly.
4. All persons, patrons, or staff who become injured or suddenly ill shall be the subject of a "Code Yellow" response. "Silent codes" shall not be used.
5. A "Code Yellow" shall exist when a person or persons are injured, or become suddenly ill, and require immediate first aid. Such person/'s are breathing and have obvious signs of circulation but may not necessarily be conscious.

PROCEDURE:

1. One person from each department shall respond to all Code Yellow pages, unless doing so will leave a high-risk patient/patron unattended.
2. Staff persons shall insure personal safety and that of any and all bystanders.
3. Staff shall arrive at the scene with vinyl gloves on hands and a pocket mask extended with the one-way valve in place.
4. Call 9-9-1-1 if the injured/ill person is unconscious, short of breath, complains of chest discomfort, is dizzy, is in pain, or is actively bleeding, or anytime there is any doubt.
5. Summon the AED and the oxygen.
6. Provide first aid care as needed.
7. Remain at the scene until excused by the supervisor on call
8. Offer to help even if not asked.
9. Complete a Patient Care Action Log
10. Remove and dispose of contaminants properly
11. Complete an Incident Report Form

PERFORMANCE IMPROVEMENT:

1. Code events will be evaluated by the response team and the *(Facility Name)* manager/director.
2. The entire process will be evaluated for timeliness, appropriateness, efficiency, and outcome.
3. Deficiencies will be noted, and methods for improvement implemented.
4. All code events will be reported to and reviewed by the physician advisory committee.

A-2c. Code Red (Fire)

(Facility Name)

POLICY AND PROCEDURE:

<table>
<tr><td colspan="1">MANUALS: (Facility Name) Safety Manual

(Facility Name) Policy & Procedures Manual</td><td colspan="2">POLICY NO.: ____</td></tr>
<tr><td>EFFECTIVE:</td><td colspan="2">SUBJECT: Code Red (Fire)</td></tr>
<tr><td>REVIEWED:</td><td colspan="2">DIVISION: (Facility Name)</td></tr>
<tr><td>REVISED:</td><td>ISSUING DEPT.:</td><td>DISTRIBUTION:

All _________ Departments</td></tr>
<tr><td>APPROVED DIRECTOR:

DATE:</td><td colspan="2">APPROVED DEPT. MANAGER:

DATE:</td></tr>
</table>

PURPOSE:

To assure safe and expedient evacuation of clients, patients, and staff in the event of a fire

POLICY:

Clarify staff responses and maximize safety to persons and property during a fire emergency.

PROCEDURE:

1. When a fire is discovered:
   A. Rescue client(s) from immediate danger.
   B. Alarm – activate fire alarm at a pull station (dial 4100 or 0 and notify the front desk of exact location of the fire, i.e., laundry room behind the dryer).
   C. Confine the fire by closing the door.
   D. Extinguish only if possible to do so without danger to yourself or the client. (Evacuate if necessary.)

E. Use stairs, not elevators.

F. Close doors, and windows, and turn off fans in the area.

G. Know where the fire is.

H. A safe area is where you have at least one set of fire doors between fire and you.

I. When a call is made to the front desk, the front desk staff will:

- Announce "CODE Red" over the emergency paging system, and give the location 3x.

- Call 9-9-1-1 and let the operator know that an alarm has sounded at *(Facility Name)* and the location of the alarm.

J. One representative from each area will respond with a fire extinguisher.

K. The on-call supervisor (MOD) will immediately respond to the scene and take charge of the situation.

L. If evacuation of the building is necessary, follow the evacuation procedure until an "all clear" is given.

2. If alarm sounds with no call to the front desk:

   A. Front desk personnel will immediately check the fire alarm panel behind the front desk.

   B. Once the area has been determined on the panel, announce "CODE RED" and the location over the emergency paging system 3x. Continue on with the regular procedure for fire. Go back to the START of procedure.

PERFORMANCE IMPROVEMENT:

1. Code events will be evaluated by the response team and the *(Facility Name)* manager/director.
2. The entire process will be evaluated for timeliness, appropriateness, efficiency, and outcome.
3. Deficiencies will be noted, and methods for improvement implemented.
4. All code events will be reported to and reviewed by the physician advisory committee.

A-2d. Code Strong (Out of Control Client/Patient)

(Facility Name)

POLICY AND PROCEDURE:

<table>
<tr><td>MANUAL: (Facility Name) Safety Manual

(Facility Name) Policy & Procedures Manual</td><td colspan="2">POLICY NO.: ____</td></tr>
<tr><td>EFFECTIVE:</td><td colspan="2">SUBJECT: Code Strong (Out of Control Client/Patient)</td></tr>
<tr><td>REVIEWED:</td><td colspan="2">DIVISION: (Facility Name)</td></tr>
<tr><td>REVISED:</td><td>ISSUING DEPT.:</td><td>DISTRIBUTION:

All _________ Departments</td></tr>
<tr><td>APPROVED DIRECTOR:

DATE:</td><td colspan="2">APPROVED DEPT. MANAGER:

DATE:</td></tr>
</table>

PURPOSE:

To provide an organized approach when a Code Strong is initiated in response to an individual (patient, member, visitor, staff) demonstrating uncontrolled, unanticipated, severely aggressive, or violent behavior which presents an imminent danger to that individual, or others

POLICY:

The (Facility Name) goal is to utilize the least restrictive method of managing a Code Strong situation while respecting the individual's rights and promoting safety. Code Strong is initiated by any employee when an individual poses a threat or becomes a danger to self or others.

PROCEDURE:

1. Initiating the Response:
   A. A call is made to the *(Facility Name)* front desk by dialing ____________ and requesting Code Strong to a specific location. The operator notifies the on-call supervisor by overhead page.

B. The on-call supervisor will make Code Strong the highest priority and immediately respond to the location. The shift supervisor will summon other team members as needed.

C. The team leader will be identified out of the responders:

- The team leader will obtain a history and make an assessment of the situation.
- The team leader will determine the initial approach to managing the situation and make appropriate assignments to the other team members.
- The team leader will be the only one to communicate with the individual.
- The team leader will direct the actions of the team.

D. If/when law enforcement support is considered necessary, the on-call supervisor will designate someone to call the phone operator who, in turn, will notify the ______________ Police Department to respond to the Code Strong location.

2. De-escalation (least restrictive):

A. Any adverse stimulant to the situation will be removed and other environmental alterations made as necessary.

B. Verbal expression by the individual will be allowed/encouraged.

C. Limits will be set on any behaviors which may jeopardize the safety of the individual or others.

D. Talk-down techniques, such as reflective listening, bargaining, and diversion, will be implemented by the team leader to redirect emotion.

E. The individual will be redirected to a safer, more appropriate environment if indicated.

F. Standard self-defense maneuvers, such as deflection of physical contact, will be employed, as necessary, to manage physical contact by the individual involved in the Code Strong.

G. Alternative interventions (comfort, environmental, and social measures) will be offered as appropriate.

H. Staff/individual ratio should be 2:1 until the individual is stable or 911 assistance arrives.

I. The immediate environment is quieted and darkened as needed.

J. The staff/patient ratio should be 1:1 until the patient is stable.

K. Physician evaluation of the individual is performed within one hour of the onset of a behavioral health-management situation.

L. The behavioral health-management flow sheet is used for documentation, as long as the situation is identified as a behavioral-health scenario.

REPORT AND PERFORMANCE IMPROVEMENT:

1. The on-call supervisor is responsible for ensuring that the post-Code Strong evaluation is completed.
2. The form will be submitted to quality management services for review of appropriateness of response and opportunities for improvement.
3. If an employee sustains an injury, an employee Injury Report form is completed.
4. If a member or visitor sustains an injury, an Event Report is completed.
5. Critical incident stress debriefing (CISD) will be arranged as needed for the team members.
6. Performance improvement, using the Focus PDCA process, will be conducted on an ongoing basis. Improvement processes will seek to identify opportunities to reduce risks associated with behavior management.

TEAM TRAINING:

Designated team members are required to complete a comprehensive training to prepare for the specific roles and techniques utilized in a Code Strong response (all team members may potentially fill any role, including team leader). Participation in practice and updates will occur periodically thereafter.

A-2e. Code Black (Bomb Threat)

(Facility Name)

POLICY AND PROCEDURE:

<table>
<tr><td colspan="1">MANUAL: (Facility Name) Safety Manual

(Facility Name) Policy & Procedures Manual</td><td colspan="2">POLICY NO.: ____</td></tr>
<tr><td>EFFECTIVE:</td><td colspan="2">SUBJECT: Code Black (Bomb Threat)</td></tr>
<tr><td>REVIEWED:</td><td colspan="2">DIVISION:</td></tr>
<tr><td>REVISED:</td><td>ISSUING DEPT.:

(Facility Name)</td><td>DISTRIBUTION:

All ________ Departments</td></tr>
<tr><td>APPROVED DIRECTOR:

DATE:</td><td colspan="2">APPROVED DEPT. MANAGER:

DATE:</td></tr>
</table>

PURPOSE:

To respond to a bomb threat

POLICY:

All staff will be familiar with Code Black procedure to ensure safe and expedient evacuation of patrons, patients and staff, and to assist with the location of the explosive device(s) when directed by the on-call supervisor.

PROCEDURE:

1. Person receiving the call/threat: Any *(Facility Name)* employee who receives a threat of an explosive device, either in person or over the telephone will observe the following procedure:
   A. Remain calm and attempt to keep the person on the line or at the *(Facility Name)* without coercion.
   B. Immediately notify nearby staff and note the exact time the call or threat is received.

C. Attempt to determine the location, description, and detonation time for the device from the perpetrator. Prolong the conversation, if possible, while evaluating the caller's voice and any background noises.

2. Nearby staff:

   A. Pull, or have another employee, pull the nearest fire alarm.

   B. Call, or have another employee immediately call the fire department (9-1-1-1) to report a bomb threat, NOT a fire.

   C. Advise the dispatcher of the nature of the call and request law enforcement at the *(Facility Name).*

   D. Have the front desk page "Code Black" three times over the emergency paging system. Speak clearly and slowly so that the words may be easily understood. The front desk should ask the on-call supervisor to verify that all departments in the *(Facility Name)* have heard the page.

   E. The on-call supervisor shall notify the ______________ administrator on duty by calling ______________ and having that individual paged. The on-call supervisor shall also immediately notify the *(Facility Name)* director.

3. Other *(Facility Name)* staff:

   A. Upon hearing a "Code Black" overhead page, all *(Facility Name)* staff will prepare to begin an immediate, but orderly evacuation of all patrons/patients.

   B. *(Facility Name)* staff shall also evacuate as directed by the on-call staff.

4. Evacuation:

   A. Staff will instruct all patrons to leave the building in an orderly fashion through the exit(s), as advised by the on-call staff. Staff should not allow patrons/patients to return to locker rooms to gather personal belongings, but should evacuate with the expectation that they may not be returning.

   B. Patrons/patients will be escorted by one or more staff designees to one of the following locations as determined by the on-call staff:

      - Northwest corner of the *(Facility Name)* north (main) parking lot. Those persons with car keys in possession may leave the premises.
      - ____
      - ____
      - *(Facility Name)* staff will relocate all children to ______________ , where they may be released to parents/guardians possessing proper identification.
      - Staff shall calmly and professionally reassure patrons/patients that the situation is under control.

5. Bomb search procedure:
   A. The on-call supervisor will assign persons, as needed, to conduct the search.
   B. The ______________ administrator and/or the *(Facility Name)* director, or in their absence, the on-call supervisor, shall assign staff and law enforcement personnel to begin the search operation. Search leaders should be designated, and persons with familiarity with specific areas should be assigned to search those areas. If the perpetrator has designated a particular location, that location should be placed under tight security until a thorough search of it has been made.
   C. The search will include, but not be limited to areas such as trash cans, closet drawers, lockers, cabinets, and conspicuous areas. Staff should be particularly aware of suspicious objects such as boxes, backpacks, canisters, etc. that appear to be unattended.
   D. Suspicious objects shall be reported to the administrator, the *(Facility Name)* director, and/or the on-call supervisor who will then advise the commanding officer of the responding safety agency; police, fire, etc.
   E. If a suspicious object is found it shall not be touched or moved.
   F. Search leaders shall report the results of their search to the on-call supervisor.
6. Evaluating the caller:
   A. Ask the caller the following questions:
      - When is the bomb set to explode?
      - Where did you place the bomb?
      - What does it look like?
      - What kind of bomb is it?
      - Why did you plant the bomb?
   B. Describe the caller's voice:
      Male____ Female____ Young____ Middle-Aged____ Elderly____
      Excited____ Calm____ Accent____ Is the voice familiar? ______

PERFORMANCE IMPROVEMENT:

1. Code events will be evaluated by the response team and the *(Facility Name)* manager/director.
2. The entire process will be evaluated for timeliness, appropriateness, efficiency, and outcome.
3. Deficiencies will be noted, and methods for improvement implemented.
4. All code events will be reported to and reviewed by the physician advisory committee.

A-2f. Code Purple (Missing Infant/Child)

(Facility Name)

POLICY AND PROCEDURE:

<table>
<tr><td colspan="1">MANUALS: (Facility Name) Manual

(Facility Name) Policy & Procedures Manual</td><td colspan="2">POLICY NO.: ____</td></tr>
<tr><td>EFFECTIVE:</td><td colspan="2">SUBJECT: Code Purple (Missing Infant/Child)</td></tr>
<tr><td>REVIEWED:</td><td colspan="2">DIVISION: (Facility Name)</td></tr>
<tr><td>REVISED:</td><td>ISSUING DEPT.:</td><td>DISTRIBUTION:

All _________ Departments</td></tr>
<tr><td>APPROVED DIRECTOR:

DATE:</td><td colspan="2">APPROVED DEPT. MANAGER:

DATE:</td></tr>
</table>

PURPOSE:

To provide a consistent procedure in the event of a missing infant/child.

POLICY:

To attempt to protect infants/children who may be in imminent danger of abduction and to locate and protect those who may have become lost while on *(Facility Name)* property. The determination of a "CODE PURPLE" will be made by the *(Facility Name)* director or the on-call supervisor at the time of the incident. DEFINITION: A "CODE PURPLE" may exist when an infant/child is physically removed or is suspected of having been physically removed from the building by someone other than his/her legal guardian or when a child has become separated from his/her legal guardian and cannot be located by said guardian by reasonable search, of common areas, and has not responded to overhead paging.

PROCEDURE:

1. In the event of the determination, by a *(Facility Name)* staff person, of a missing infant/child, or the suspicion thereof:

A. The on-call supervisor will be notified immediately by the staff person or a designee that a "CODE PURPLE" may exist. The on-call supervisor will then respond immediately to the front desk, recognizing that TIME IS OF THE ESSENCE!

B. The front desk will page once on the general overhead and once on the emergency paging system for the missing child, (when age appropriate) to report to the front desk. If no response occurs, the front desk will then, at the discretion of the On Call Supervisor:

  - Call 911, staying on the line to provide pertinent information.
  - The on-call supervisor will direct the front desk to page "Code Purple," using the emergency paging system. The page will be announced three times, followed by a description of the missing child, including name, age, gender, and clothing description.
  - The on-call supervisor will notify the *(Facility Name)* director that a "CODE PURPLE" exists.

C. Staff members will close all exits to the building. No children fitting the description of the "CODE PURPLE" in question, and no adult/s accompanied by children of said description will be allowed to leave the building until satisfactory identification has been obtained. Any discrepancies will be referred to the on-call supervisor. Staff members will attempt, using body positioning and/or dialogue to prevent the child in question or an adult accompanied by a child meeting the description of the "CODE PURPLE" from leaving the building. Staff members are to avoid injury to themselves or others at all costs.

D. The on-call supervisor will act as contact person for law enforcement. The on-call supervisor will coordinate the search, when indicated, from the front desk.

E. Other staff will search the building for the missing child, beginning in their respective departments, including, but not limited to, all rooms, laundry and utility rooms, washers and dryers, second floor rooms, patio, garbage cans, cupboards, and refrigerators.

F. Each department will notify the on-call supervisor of the results of the search in the respective department.

G. The on-call supervisor will contact social services/pastoral care to provide support for the parents.

H. The front desk will announce "Code Purple all clear" over the emergency paging system at the appropriate time.

2. Staff response in other departments:

A. Appropriate departments will secure entrances/exits/stairwells.

B. See step (E) above

C. Pool staff will clear pools of all occupants and gather them in the area adjacent to the towel and blanket storage cabinet at the south exit until the announcement "Code Purple all clear" is given.

D. All staff will challenge/detain all persons with infants/children. See paragraph 2.F. Proof of identity will be required, and no one will be allowed to leave the building with an infant/child until proper identification is produced.

E. Staff will <u>request</u> to check backpacks, shopping bags, or other possible areas of concealment for persons exiting the building.

F. Security of exits will be maintained until "Code Purple all clear" is announced overhead.

3. If this is a witnessed abduction, the witness/staff person will:

   A. Follow steps described in paragraphs 1. A-C above.

   B. Attempt to retrieve the infant/child from the abductor and return him/her to the front desk. Do not endanger yourself or the child in doing so. If the abductor leaves the facility, and staff is available, one staff person should follow the abductor at a safe distance and speed. Before doing so, the staff member must notify another staff member of his/her departure from the building. Take a cellular phone or two-way radio if available. Get a description of the abductor and the vehicle. Note the direction the vehicle's description, direction of travel, and license plate number if possible. Telephone the on-call supervisor with this information.

PERFORMANCE IMPROVEMENT:

1. Code events will be evaluated by the response team and the *(Facility Name)* manager/director.
2. The entire process will be evaluated for timeliness, appropriateness, efficiency, and outcome.
3. Deficiencies will be noted, and methods for improvement implemented.
4. All code events will be reported to and reviewed by the physician advisory committee.

Appendix A-3
AED & CPR Training Plan

AEDs and rescue equipment are only as effective as the people trained to use them. Quality training and continued responder practice are essential to AED and emergency response program success.

At a minimum, an AED program training plan should address the following:

- Selection of responders
- Initial Training
- Recurring Training

SELECTION OF RESPONDERS:

AED program responders come from all walks of life, and do not necessarily require any particular background. At a minimum, responders should have a desire to help others. Responders should be able-bodied, and capable of physically performing the skills of CPR and AED.

Carefully consider your Site Survey (Appendix B-2e), and select individuals who are likely to be regularly present and able to respond when an emergency arises. Consider all hours of operation of your organization, and different "shifts" of people that may be present. Some organizations require multiple groups of responders to be trained. Others require that all staff undergo CPR and AED training.

INITIAL TRAINING:

Most organizations conduct a training program for AED responders that teaches cardiopulmonary resuscitation (CPR) and AED use (e.g. Heartsaver AED or higher level). Additional modules, such as infant/child CPR, and first aid may be considered, depending on your organization's needs. Completion of most training programs results in a #1 or #2 certification for responders. Some states require current certification as a condition of AED use.

There are a variety of training options for AED program responders, from a variety of sources. Most training courses are traditional instructor-led classes that are conducted at your organization. Where this is not practical, some self-guided training programs may be used. Whenever possible, responders should have the opportunity to practice the use of the exact AED model owned by their organization.

Although a variety of organizations purport to offer CPR and AED training programs, American Heart Association training programs are widely regarded at the "gold standard" of emergency-care training. The American Heart Association is the scientific body that routinely reviews the science of resuscitation and sets the generally accepted professional standards for emergency cardiovascular care in the United States. Its training programs closely follow these guidelines and reflect the latest in resuscitation science.

RECURRING TRAINING:

Studies have shown that resuscitation skills decline precipitously in as little as six months. As with any skill, practice makes perfect. It is essential that responders practice skills regularly to remain proficient and confident in their skills. At a minimum, responders should repeat (or re-certify) their training every one to two years, as recommended by the training organization. Additionally, periodic skill refreshers, or response "drills", are an effective way to keep responder skills sharp.

TRACKING & MAINTENANCE:

Most modern AEDs do not require frequent routine maintenance. Because care requirements can vary significantly from model to model, you should be sure to familiarize yourself with the manufacturer's recommendations for the AED that you own, or intend to own.

PADS & BATTERIES:

Fortunately, most AEDs found in AED programs are not frequently used. Typically, an AED that is not regularly used will require replacement of its *batteries* and *pads* every few years. Defibrillator pads contain a water-based gel that will dry out over time, and render the pads unusable. Most pads have expiration dates indicated on them.

SELF-TESTING:

Most AEDs employ some degree of self-testing to regularly check the AED and detect common problems, such as a low battery. The AED may notify you to a problem with either audible or visual indicators.

TRACKING:

It is essential that items such as pads and batteries are kept current to ensure that the AED is ready for use. Some method of tracking the location of AEDs, the accessories with them, and the expiration of pads and batteries is essential. This may be accomplished in conjunction with a medical oversight program.

REGULAR INSPECTIONS:

Although most AEDs do not require much routine maintenance, a schedule of routine inspections should be conducted to ensure that the AED is present, in working order, pads and batteries are unexpired, and all accessories are present. Recommendations for inspection intervals vary by AED and by type of organization, but many AED programs inspect equipment on a monthly basis.

Appendix A-4
Sample Safety-Inspection Program

THE SUMMIT
Medical Fitness Center
205 Sunnyview Lane • Kalispell, MT 59901
406-751-4100 • SUMMITHEALTHCENTER.com

Formal periodic standardized safety inspections are an important part of an accident-prevention program. Safety inspections are a formal review of the work environment, conducted to identify physical conditions or employee actions that may result in employee or member injuries. The desired result is to make changes in the work environment or employee behavior prior to an accident occurring.

The inspection process provides a means to review the work process performed by the employees to determine if the workers are effectively following the safety requirements of their work. Inspections are performed to assist in the effective control of loss producing activity. The more likelihood of a severe injury occurring or probability of a high frequency of minor injuries occurring would require a higher frequency of inspection. When the inspection process identifies substandard items, corrective action must be forthcoming, or the credibility of the safety effort may come into question.

Inspections allow for the general review of operations to determine the effectiveness of the overall safety program. High numbers of substandard conditions or practices may be symptomatic of the need for management action.

FREQUENCY:

1. Department inspections will be performed on a monthly basis in each department, location. These inspections will be documented using the attached inspection report. All monthly inspections must be completed and returned to the operations manager by the 15th of each month.
2. Facility inspections will be performed on a quarterly basis by the operations manager. These inspections will be documented using the attached inspection report.

COMPLIANCE:

1. It is the responsibility of the Summit staff to submit work order requests. Copies of the request are to be maintained by the operations manager.

2. Any repeated non-compliance safety issue will be addressed by the operations manager for methods to make the facility compliant.
3. The goal of the inspection and audit process is to provide a safe environment while administrating accountability.

Center Manager's Monthly Safety Inspection

Location: The Summit

Month: ______________________ Date Submitted: ______________________

Have all employees received their safety orientation?	Yes	No	n/a
Did all new employees receive a safety orientation as part of the new hire process?	Yes	No	n/a
Were all daily safety audits completed?	Yes	No	n/a
Were all unsafe conditions corrected at the time?	Yes	No	n/a
Were all weekly safety audits completed?	Yes	No	n/a
Were all unsafe conditions corrected at the time?	Yes	No	n/a
Were there any member injuries this month?	Yes	No	n/a
If yes, were the event-report forms completed?	Yes	No	n/a
Are code drills preformed monthly?	Yes	No	n/a

How many employees did you personally speak to this month regarding safety issues? ______

Please list their names below:

1. ______________________ 2. ______________________

3. ______________________ 4. ______________________

5. ______________________ 6. ______________________

Monthly Facility Safety Inspection

Facility: The Summit

Date: ______________________ Time: ______________

Auditor: ______________________ Title: ______________ Score: ______________

General Safety

Have all employees received general safety training (fire, earthquake, VDT's, lifting, emergency evacuation, etc)?	Yes	No	n/a
Are all employees familiar with the use of the MSDS?	Yes	No	n/a
Have all employees received proper training in how to operate the equipment they are required to use?	Yes	No	n/a
Have all employees been trained in how to protect themselves from the hazards identified in their work area?	Yes	No	n/a
Are the OSHA information poster, the workmen's compensation bulletin, and other mandated signs posted?	Yes	No	n/a
Are glass doors and partitions marked at eye level and in good condition?	Yes	No	n/a
Are alarm systems working properly and is access restricted?	Yes	No	n/a

Score = Number of YES Responses x 1

Monthly Facility Safety Inspection *continued*

Facility: The Summit

Date: ______________________ Time: ______________

Auditor: ______________________ Title: ______________ Score: ____________

Fitness Area

Are stairs, ramps, floors, and aisles clean and free of obstructions?	Yes	No	n/a
Are floors free of defects and other tripping hazards?	Yes	No	n/a
Are equipment and materials placed in racks or otherwise stored safely?	Yes	No	n/a
Is supervision present when necessary and is properly trained?	Yes	No	n/a
Are the floors free from loose threshold plates, loose tiles, open carpet seams, buckles, and other tripping hazards?	Yes	No	n/a
Is equipment inspected to assure it remains in good condition free from metal fatigue, fabric damage or breaks and similar defects that may compromise equipment?	Yes	No	n/a
Are weights stacked appropriately?	Yes	No	n/a
Are mirrors clean & free of cracks?	Yes	No	n/a
Is an emergency light source provided?	Yes	No	n/a
Is the AED in good working order?	Yes	No	n/a

Score = Number of YES Responses x 1

Monthly Facility Safety Inspection *continued*

Facility: The Summit

Date: ______________________ Time: ______________

Auditor:______________________ Title: ______________ Score: ____________

Building & Grounds

Are exterior walkways and parking lots are free of tripping hazards?	Yes	No	n/a
Are stairways, parking areas, sidewalks, and yards well lit and free of obstructions?	Yes	No	n/a
Are curb edges clearly identified by means of contrasting colors?	Yes	No	n/a
Are grounds free of debris and litter?	Yes	No	n/a
Are the sprinkler heads positioned so that they do not present a tripping hazard?	Yes	No	n/a
Are hazardous areas properly posted?	Yes	No	n/a
Are trees and shrubs properly trimmed?	Yes	No	n/a
Is the fencing in good repair with no sharp projections?	Yes	No	n/a
Are entrances – all doors, steps, carpets/mats, & runners–in good condition?	Yes	No	n/a
Are electrical outlets & fuse boxes properly secured, labeled & grounded?	Yes	No	n/a
Are all emergence lights in good working order tested monthly?	Yes	No	n/a
Are all exterior lights in good working order?	Yes	No	n/a

Score = Number of YES Responses x 1

Monthly Facility Safety Inspection *continued*

Facility: The Summit

Date: ______________________ Time: ______________

Auditor: ______________________ Title: ______________ Score: ____________

Office & Break Rooms

Are floors free of defects and other tripping hazards?	Yes	No	n/a
Are chairs, equipment and materials placed/stored in racks or other wise stored safely?	Yes	No	n/a
Is lost property in a secure location?	Yes	No	n/a
Are memorandums and bulletins posted and available to staff?	Yes	No	n/a
Is the area clean and properly maintained?	Yes	No	n/a
Are appliances operational and free of water and other hazards?	Yes	No	n/a
Is the doorway free of clutter?	Yes	No	n/a
Is material stored properly?	Yes	No	n/a
Is the entrance signed for staff use only?	Yes	No	n/a
Is an emergency light source provided?	Yes	No	n/a

Score = Number of YES Responses x 1

Monthly Facility Safety Inspection *continued*

Facility: The Summit

Date: ______________________ Time: ______________

Auditor:______________________ Title: ______________ Score: ____________

Locker Rooms

Are floor mats free of defects and other tripping hazards?	Yes	No	n/a
Are floors in good repair and not slippery?	Yes	No	n/a
Are mirrors & tiles clean and free of chips & cracks?	Yes	No	n/a
Is the locker room clean and orderly?	Yes	No	n/a
Are benches & lockers clean and free of hazards?	Yes	No	n/a
Are toilets & showers clean and free of hazards?	Yes	No	n/a
Is an emergency light source provided?	Yes	No	n/a

Score = Number of YES Responses x 1

Monthly Facility Safety Inspection *continued*

Facility: The Summit

Date: ______________________ Time: ______________

Auditor: ______________________ Title: ______________ Score: ____________

Steam/Sauna Rooms

Are floors free of defects and other tripping hazards?	Yes	No	n/a
Are floors in good repair and not slippery?	Yes	No	n/a
Are tiles clean and free of chips & cracks?	Yes	No	n/a
Are temperature standards being followed?	Yes	No	n/a
Are benches secure and free of hazards?	Yes	No	n/a
Are heat elements labeled as high temperature?	Yes	No	n/a
Are signs dictating rules of use posted?	Yes	No	n/a
Are all lights in working?	Yes	No	n/a
Is an emergency light source provided?	Yes	No	n/a

Score = Number of YES Responses x 1

Monthly Facility Safety Inspection *continued*

Facility: The Summit

Date: ______________________ Time: ______________

Auditor: ______________________ Title: ______________ Score: ____________

Aquatics/Pool Area

Is the area properly signed?	Yes	No	n/a
Are aquatics rescue equipment and materials placed in racks or otherwise stored safely and readily available in emergency?	Yes	No	n/a
Is supervision properly trained and present when necessary?	Yes	No	n/a
Are pool decks in good repair, free of hazards, clean, and with no standing water?	Yes	No	n/a
Is furniture clean, free of damage, and stored properly?	Yes	No	n/a
Are water quality tests performed?	Yes	No	n/a
Are pool chemical areas properly ventilated & secure?	Yes	No	n/a
Are chemical areas equipped with eyewash stations and properly maintained?	Yes	No	n/a
Are emergency exits "entrance-secured" and operational?	Yes	No	n/a
Is an emergency light source provided?	Yes	No	n/a

Score = Number of YES Responses x 1

Monthly Facility Safety Inspection *continued*

Facility: The Summit

Date: ______________________ Time: ______________

Auditor: ______________________ Title: ______________ Score: ______________

Basketball/Racquetball Courts & Studios

Are floors free of defects and other tripping hazards?	Yes	No	n/a
Are materials and equipment placed in or on racks or otherwise stored safely?	Yes	No	n/a
Are exit routes clearly identified, marked and illuminated by a reliable light source?	Yes	No	n/a
Is the area properly supervised during programs and activity times?	Yes	No	n/a
Is an emergency light source provided?	Yes	No	n/a
Are storage rooms closed and locked?	Yes	No	n/a
Are all safety nets in good condition?	Yes	No	n/a

Score = Number of YES Responses x 1

Monthly Facility Safety Inspection *continued*

Facility: The Summit

Date: ______________________ Time: ______________

Auditor: ______________________ Title: ______________ Score: ______________

Conference Rooms

Are floors free of defects and other tripping hazards?	Yes	No	n/a
Are chairs, equipment, and materials placed in racks or otherwise stored safely?	Yes	No	n/a
Are tables and chairs and in good condition?	Yes	No	n/a
Are exit routes clearly identified, marked, and illuminated by a reliable light source?	Yes	No	n/a
Are appropriate set-up procedures posted?	Yes	No	n/a
Is an emergency light source provided?	Yes	No	n/a

Score = Number of YES Responses x 1

Monthly Facility Safety Inspection *continued*

Facility: The Summit

Date: ____________________ Time: ____________

Auditor: ____________________ Title: ____________ Score: ____________

Climbing Structure

Are harnesses properly maintained?	Yes	No	n/a
Are shoes properly maintained?	Yes	No	n/a
Do carabineers lock properly?	Yes	No	n/a
Are all Grigri's in good working condition?	Yes	No	n/a
Are space requirements being maintained in the "fall area"?	Yes	No	n/a
Are holds and the wall clean and secure?	Yes	No	n/a
Are storage cabinets closed and locked?	Yes	No	n/a
Are staff able to observe the wall during their performance of duties?	Yes	No	n/a
Are members being trained on safety and proper use of the wall and equipment?	Yes	No	n/a
Are liability waivers being filed prior to use?	Yes	No	n/a
Are staff trained to inspect equipment and use of the wall?	Yes	No	n/a

Score = Number of YES Responses x 1

Monthly Facility Safety Inspection *continued*

Facility: The Summit

Date: ______________________ Time: ______________

Auditor: ______________________ Title: ______________ Score: ____________

Tyke Town

Do staff verify parents and children during check-in & out and are the child sign-in logs accurate & properly maintained?	Yes	No	n/a
Do all electrical outlets have protective coverings?	Yes	No	n/a
Are surface (floors, walls, tables etc.) areas and rooms clean and free of hazards (scissors, sharp objects, cords etc.)?	Yes	No	n/a
Are all activity areas and bathrooms orderly, well lit, and clean?	Yes	No	n/a
Are fire panic alarms secured with safety covers?	Yes	No	n/a
Are all trash and/or diaper receptacles emptied regularly?	Yes	No	n/a
Are children constantly monitor/supervised in a manageable ratio?	Yes	No	n/a
Are both indoor and outdoor play structures sturdy, in proper working order, and properly maintained?	Yes	No	n/a
Are toys stored safely off the floor and properly kept clean and in good condition?	Yes	No	n/a
Are entrance/exit doors secure, properly alarmed and tested?	Yes	No	n/a
Is an emergency light source provided?	Yes	No	n/a

Score = Number of YES Responses x 1

Monthly Facility Safety Inspection *continued*

Facility: The Summit

Date: ______________________ Time: ______________

Auditor: ______________________ Title: ______________ Score: ____________

S.P.A.R.K. Zone

Do staff verify children during check-in & out and are the child sign-in logs accurate & properly maintained?	Yes	No	n/a
Are surface (floors, walls, tables etc.) areas and rooms clean and free of hazards (scissors, sharp objects, cords etc.)?	Yes	No	n/a
Are all activity areas and bathrooms orderly, well lit, and clean?	Yes	No	n/a
Are all trash receptacles emptied regularly?	Yes	No	n/a
Are children constantly monitor/supervised in a manageable ratio?	Yes	No	n/a
Are toys and games stored safely off the floor and properly kept clean and in good condition?	Yes	No	n/a
Is an emergency light source provided?	Yes	No	n/a

Score = Number of YES Responses x 1

Monthly Facility Safety Inspection *continued*

Facility: The Summit

Date: ______________________ Time: ______________

Auditor: ______________________ Title: ______________ Score: ______________

Tennis Courts

Are courts free of defects and other tripping hazards?	Yes	No	n/a
Are courts clean and well lit?	Yes	No	n/a
Are all trash receptacles emptied regularly?	Yes	No	n/a
Are tennis nets in good condition?	Yes	No	n/a
Are court divider nets in good condition?	Yes	No	n/a
Are tables and chairs and in good condition?	Yes	No	n/a
Is an emergency light source provided?	Yes	No	n/a
Is equipment stored safely off the floor and properly kept clean and in good condition?	Yes	No	n/a
Is the ball machine in good working condition?	Yes	No	n/a
Are all backstop nets in good condition?	Yes	No	n/a

Score = Number of YES Responses x 1

Monthly Facility Safety Inspection *continued*

Facility: The Summit

Date: ______________________ Time: ______________

Auditor: ______________________ Title: ______________ Score: ____________

Hazardous Materials & Chemical Storage

Are all chemicals used in the area stored in safe containers, inaccessible to members?	Yes	No	n/a
Are chemical storage areas secure and well lit?	Yes	No	n/a
Are chemical containers clearly and accurately labeled?	Yes	No	n/a
Are chemical disposal procedures being followed and enforced?	Yes	No	n/a
Are MSDS information sheets current?	Yes	No	n/a
Is hazardous material information/MSDS readily available?	Yes	No	n/a
Are staff being trained on and properly understand MSDS content sheets?	Yes	No	n/a

Score = Number of YES Responses x 1

Monthly Facility Safety Inspection *continued*

Facility: The Summit

Date: ______________________ Time: ______________

Auditor:______________________ Title: ______________ Score: ____________

Emergency & Fire Safety

Are exit routes clearly identified, marked, and illuminated by a reliable light source?	Yes	No	n/a
Are emergency exit signs lit and tested monthly?	Yes	No	n/a
Are there at least two exits provided from building interiors?	Yes	No	n/a
Do the exit doors swings in the direction of exit travel?	Yes	No	n/a
Is an emergency light source provided and tested monthly?	Yes	No	n/a
Are ceilings and wall surfaces on escape routes kept free from combustible, decorative, or functional materials?	Yes	No	n/a
Are fire extinguishers present, readily accessible, and operational (properly serviced & tagged) checked monthly?	Yes	No	n/a
Are fire extinguishers properly secured & mounted?	Yes	No	n/a
Are fire extinguishers mounted in such a manner that the top of the extinguisher is not more than 5′ above the floor?	Yes	No	n/a
Are first-aid kits adequate for facility and properly maintained with supplies?	Yes	No	n/a
Are first-aid kits readily available?	Yes	No	n/a
Are fire-exit alarms operational?	Yes	No	n/a

Score = Number of YES Responses x 1

Monthly Safety Inspection Recap

Facility: The Summit

Month: ______________________

Section	**Description**	**Score**
1	General Safety	________
2	Fitness Area	________
3	Building & Grounds	________
4	Office & Break Rooms	________
5	Locker Rooms	________
6	Steam/Sauna Rooms	________
7	Aquatics/Pool Area	________
8	Basketball/Racquet Ball Courts & Studios	________
9	Conference Rooms	________
10	Climbing Structure	________
11	Tyke Town	________
12	S.P.A.R.K. Zone	________
13	Tennis	________
14	Hazardous Materials & Chemical Storage	________
15	Emergency & Fire Safety	________

Total Monthly Audit Score: ________ *Total possible 136*

Deficiencies and Corrective Action

List any problems found and corrective action taken:

____

____

____

Appendix A-5
Sample Job Descriptions

A-5a Position Title: Facility Director/General Manager

Position Summary:

The general manager is accountable for the overall financial and operational success of the facility. The general manager is responsible for the recruitment, selection, and development of the employee team, and the leadership of that team in a manner that will drive achievement of the facility's annual business plan and budgetary goals.

Essential Accountabilities & Functions:

- To be accountable for the development of the facility's annual business plan and budget (operational and capital), along with monitoring actual performance to ensure achievement of the business plan and budget targets
- To be accountable for the selection and development of the facility's employee team and providing an environment that ensures that the employees work as a team in achieving the facility's goals
- To be accountable for fostering an environment that embraces the culture of the facility and creates personalized experiences for each user
- To be accountable for overseeing the daily operations of the facility
- To be accountable for the facility's quality-management program

Specific Job Accountabilities:

- Develop the annual business plan and and associated capital and operational budgets.
- Oversee the financial activities of the facility in a manner that will bring about achievement of the facility's financial goals, including driving revenues, managing expenses, and achieving bottom-line performance numbers.

- Recruit, select, develop, educate, and lead the employee team, including conducting regular meetings for the staff and performing regular (e.g., annual) performance reviews on all direct reports, per organizational policy.
- Serve as the facility's public-relations voice by getting involved in the local community, including serving on local boards and committees, speaking to community groups, and supporting community-based healthcare activities.
- Oversee the day-to-day operations of the facility, including opening and closing of the facility, as may be needed.
- Maximize the safety of all facility users by overseeing the facility's safety and emergency-response programs. Ensure that all staff maintain current training for safety and emergency response.
- Oversee all activities of the facility's quality-management and performance-improvement programs.
- Serve as a role model for the employees, including performing any necessary job responsibilities, as may be required to ensure that the facility delivers upon its MFA commitment to excellence.

Reporting Relationships:

- Reports to: Owner or corporate administrator
- Directly supervises: All department heads
- Indirectly supervises: All frontline staff

Work Experience:

- Minimum of three year's experience in a supervisory role within the medical fitness or health/wellness industry
- Minimum of one year's experience as a fitness center or medical fitness center manager

Education:

- College degree in health/wellness, fitness, or a related field

Certification/License:

- Certification from a NCCA-accredited health/fitness certification organization preferred, but not required
- AED/CPR certification

*Adapted from Stephen J. Tharrett and James A. Peterson. *Fitness Management (2nd Edition)*. Monterey, CA: Healthy Learning; 2008.

A-5b Position Title: Medical Director

Position Summary:

The medical director is responsible for providing medical guidance to the facility and its associated departments and program offerings

Essential Accountabilities & Functions:

- To provide medical guidance for the facility and associated departments and programs
- To be responsible for reviewing and approving patient-care policies, procedures, and patient-care standards and all emergency-response policies and procedures
- To serve as a physician leader in assuring high clinical standards in facility departments and/or programs through participation in standard-of-care reviews and process-improvement activities
- To chair the physician (or medical) advisory committee

Specific Job Accountabilities:

- Provide guidance and direction to the facility to foster stronger relations with the community, including recommending patient and client satisfaction measurements in the delivery of clinical services and programs.
- Cooperate with the facility in the effective management of the facility.
- Serve as a liaison between the facility and the medical staff of the hospital(s) with which the facility has a cooperative relationship.
- Participate in the development of the facility's strategic plan and associated operating and capital budgets.
- Assist in preparing for and responding to surveys, inspections, and reviews by accrediting, licensing, and regulatory entities.
- Serve as an educational resource within the facility by participating in lectures, presentations, recommending guest speakers, and conducting staff training on specific topics.

Reporting Relationships:

- Reports to: The director/general manager of the facility
- Indirectly reports to: N/A
- Directly supervises: N/A
- Indirectly supervises: N/A

*Adapted from Stephen J. Tharrett and James A. Peterson. *Fitness Management (2nd Edition).* Monterey, CA: Healthy Learning; 2008.

Work Experience:

- Minimum of two years post-residency experience in a hospital or clinical setting

Education:

- Medical degree from an accredited program

Certification/License:

- Licensure by state medical board

*Adapted from Stephen J. Tharrett and James A. Peterson. *Fitness Management (2nd Edition).* Monterey, CA: Healthy Learning; 2008.

A-5c Position Title: Fitness Manager/Director/Supervisor

Position Summary:

The fitness manager/director is accountable for the facility's fitness and group exercise programs and, in particular, for achieving the budgeted financial performance of the fitness department.

Essential Accountabilities & Functions:

- To oversee the development of the annual business plan and financial targets for the fitness department, along with monitoring actual financial performance of key revenue and expense areas to help ensure achievement of the business plan and financial-plan targets
- To be accountable for the recruitment, selection, and development of the facility's fitness and group-exercise staff and for insuring that the employees work as a team in achieving the department's and facility's goals
- To be accountable for ensuring scientifically and medically sound fitness programming
- To be accountable for providing a safe environment for all facility users and staff
- To respond to all emergency situations per facility policy and procedures
- To be accountable for fostering a fitness environment that leads to user satisfaction
- To be accountable for making sure that every user who is on the fitness floor is served in a manner that ensures them of a memorable experience in the facility
- To be accountable for the overall condition and cleanliness of the fitness and exercise equipment and areas in the facility

Specific Job Accountabilities:

- Develop the department's annual business plan and financial targets.
- Manage the daily, weekly, and monthly revenue activities of the department, so as to enable the facility to achieve its fitness-revenue target objectives.
- Oversee the financial activities of the department in a manner that will bring about achievement of the department's financial goals, including driving revenues and managing department expenses.
- Oversee and monitor new user screenings and orientations and directing users into activities that will engage them in a long-term fitness program. This step includes daily, weekly, monthly, and YTD monitoring.

*Adapted from Stephen J. Tharrett and James A. Peterson. *Fitness Management (2nd Edition).* Monterey, CA: Healthy Learning; 2008.

- Recruit, select, develop, educate, and lead the fitness and group-exercise team, including conducting regular meetings, providing continuing-education activities, and performing regular (e.g., annual) performance reviews on all direct reports.
- Establish relationships with the users by engaging these individuals with a service attitude while they are on the fitness floor.
- Oversee the care of the fitness areas, including inspecting the equipment, making sure the proper preventative maintenance for equipment is addressed, replacing and updating equipment, as needed, and otherwise ensuring that the fitness area is clean, well-maintained, and safe for the users.
- Oversee the day-to-day operations of the department, including completing all necessary administrative functions required by the facility.
- Serve as a role model for the fitness staff, including performing any necessary job responsibilities as may be required to ensure that the facility delivers upon its MFA commitment to excellence.

Reporting Relationships:

- Reports to: Facility's director/general manager
- Indirectly reports to: N/A
- Directly supervises: Fitness instructors, personal trainers, and group-exercise staff
- Indirectly supervises: Housecleaning staff

Work Experience:

- Minimum of one year's experience in a supervisory role within the fitness industry
- Minimum of three year's experience as a personal trainer or fitness instructor

Education:

- Bachelor's degree in exercise science, fitness, health, kinesiology, or recreation
- Master's degree/graduate work in fitness or a related field preferred

Certification/License:

- Certification as a personal trainer, fitness instructor, or conditioning specialist from a NCCA-accredited certification organization (e.g., ACE, ACSM, NASM, NSCA)
- Secondary certification in a fitness specialty area preferred, but not required
- AED/CPR certification

*Adapted from Stephen J. Tharrett and James A. Peterson. *Fitness Management (2nd Edition).* Monterey, CA: Healthy Learning; 2008.

A-5d Position Title: Fitness Instructor

Position Summary:

The position of fitness instructor is responsible for providing a safe and effective exercise environment for facility users by supervising individual exercise programs, educating the individuals who are exercising, and establishing a personalized program of exercise for each user.

Essential Accountabilities & Functions:

- To provide supervision of the exercise and fitness areas of the facility, including assisting users with their exercise and fitness program
- To evaluate each user's fitness needs and provide the appropriate exercise program for meeting those needs, including providing personal instruction if necessary
- To connect users to other users through ongoing contact with the individuals and the promotion of the facility's activities

Specific Job Accountabilities:

- Conduct new user fitness assessments and/or orientations in accordance with facility standards.
- Provide fitness floor supervision, including connecting with each user on the fitness floor.
- Create personalized exercise/fitness programs for users, including providing personal coaching and education of each individual.
- Ensure that all exercise areas and equipment are in safe and effective working condition, including a level of cleanliness that is maintained to facility standards.
- Assist with any required job activity of the department, as may be needed, so as to ensure users are always served in accordance with the facility's overall service philosophy.
- Conduct oneself at all times in a manner of professionalism that aligns with the values, philosophies, and standards of the facility.
- Attend all scheduled employee meetings.
- Respond to all emergency situations according to facility policy and procedures.

Reporting Relationships:

- Reports to: Fitness director
- Directly supervises: N/A
- Indirectly supervises: N/A

*Adapted from Stephen J. Tharrett and James A. Peterson. *Fitness Management (2nd Edition).* Monterey, CA: Healthy Learning; 2008.

Work Experience:

- Minimum of one year's experience in the medical fitness or health/wellness industry preferred

Education:

- College certificate or associate's degree in exercise science, health/wellness, fitness, recreation, or a related field; bachelor's degree preferred

Certification/License:

- Certification from a NCCA-accredited fitness organization, such as ACSM, ACE, NSCA, NASM, etc.
- Certification in AED/CPR

*Adapted from Stephen J. Tharrett and James A. Peterson. *Fitness Management (2nd Edition).* Monterey, CA: Healthy Learning; 2008.

A-5e Position Title: Personal Trainer

Position Summary:

The personal trainer is responsible for providing users of the facility with a personalized fitness and healthy lifestyle program, which includes assessment of their fitness needs and then prescribing an exercise/lifestyle plan that will assist the users in achieving their goals.

Essential Accountabilities & Functions:

- To greet each user and guest who enters the fitness floor with an engaging and enthusiastic attitude and ensure that they get to know that individual by name.
- To provide users with a personalized fitness program, including the development of the fitness program, instruction in the execution of the program, and supporting the users in adhering to the prescribed program.
- To achieve monthly personal training and related revenue program targets, as established by the facility.
- To provide support in properly maintaining and cleaning the fitness equipment and fitness floor.
- To maximize the safety of each user by assisting in appropriate fitness area/equipment instruction/supervision and appropriate exercise program development, based on each individual's health and fitness condition.

Specific Job Accountabilities:

- Greet each user and guest by name when they are on the fitness floor, including establishing a relationship with each individual you greeted.
- Conduct new user assessments and orientations.
- Promote the facility's personal training and related fitness services to users and guests.
- Provide personal training and any related personal instruction for users and guests appropriate to each individual's health and fitness status.
- Assist in facilitating personal contact between users when they are on the exercise floor.
- Assist with the preventative maintenance and cleaning of the fitness equipment.
- Assist with the cleaning and care of the fitness area.
- Willingly step in and assist with other facility service responsibilities, including teaching group-fitness classes, as may be required to ensure that the facility delivers upon its MFA commitment to excellence.

*Adapted from Stephen J. Tharrett and James A. Peterson. *Fitness Management (2nd Edition).* Monterey, CA: Healthy Learning; 2008.

Reporting Relationships:

- Reports to: Personal-training supervisor and/or fitness manager/director
- Indirectly reports to: Fitness director

Work Experience:

- Minimum of one year's experience as a personal trainer and/or fitness instructor preferred.

Education:

- College certificate or associate's degree; bachelor's degree in exercise science or related field preferred.

Certification/License:

- Certification as a fitness instructor and/or personal trainer from a NCAA-accredited organization, such as ACE, ACSM, NASM, NSCA, etc.
- Successful completion of the facility's internal training requirements within 90 days of employment
- Level-two personal trainers must show evidence of having earned a second nationally accredited fitness certification
- AED/CPR certification

*Adapted from Stephen J. Tharrett and James A. Peterson. *Fitness Management (2nd Edition).* Monterey, CA: Healthy Learning; 2008.

A-5f Position Title: Aquatics Director

Position Summary:

The aquatics director is accountable for the programs and activities conducted in the facility's aquatics and pool areas and, also, for helping ensure that the budgeted financial performance of the aquatics department is achieved.

Essential Accountabilities & Functions:

- To oversee the development of the annual business plan and financial targets for the aquatics department, along with monitoring actual financial performance of key revenue and expense areas to ensure achievement of the business plan and financial-plan targets
- To be accountable for the recruitment, selection, and development of the aquatics and pool area staff and for insuring that the employees work as a team in achieving the department's and facility's goals
- To oversees departmental staff scheduling
- To be accountable for fostering an aquatics environment that maximizes safety and leads to user satisfaction
- To be accountable for making sure that every user who is in the aquatics and pool areas is served in a manner that ensures that individual of having a memorable experience in the facility
- To be accountable for the overall condition and cleanliness of the aquatics and pool equipment and areas in the facility

Specific Job Accountabilities:

- Develop the department's annual business plan and financial targets.
- Manage the daily, weekly, and monthly revenue and operational activities of the department, so as to enable the facility to achieve its aquatics performance and revenue targets.
- Maintain written policy/procedure manual for the aquatics area(s).
- Recruit, select, develop, educate, and lead the team of aquatics and pool employees, including conducting regular meetings, providing continuing education activities, and performing regular (e.g., annual) performance reviews on all direct reports.
- Ensure that all aquatics staff are appropriately trained and provided with regular practice for responding to water-related emergencies according to facility policy and procedures.
- Establish relationships with users by engaging them with a service attitude while they are in the aquatics and pool areas.

*Adapted from Stephen J. Tharrett and James A. Peterson. *Fitness Management (2nd Edition).* Monterey CA: Healthy Learning; 2008.

- Oversee proper maintenance and monitoring of the pool environment to ensure that it meets all required local health codes and user needs, a factor that includes monitoring and balancing water chemistry, monitoring and maintaining pool temperature, and monitoring and maintaining the cleanliness of the pool.
- Oversee the care of the aquatics areas, including inspecting the equipment, making sure the proper preventative maintenance for equipment is addressed, replacing and updating equipment, as needed, and otherwise ensuring that the aquatics and pool areas are clean, well-maintained, and safe for the users, including filter-room equipment, heaters, and pool surfaces.
- Oversee the day-to-day operations of the department, including completing all necessary administrative functions required by the facility.
- Serve as a role model for the aquatics and pool staff, including performing any necessary job responsibilities as may be required to ensure that the facility delivers upon its MFA commitment to excellence.

Reporting Relationships:

- Reports to: The director/general manager of the facility
- Indirectly reports to: Fitness director
- Directly supervises: Aquatics instructors, lifeguards, and pool-related, group-exercise staff
- Indirectly supervises: N/A

Work Experience:

- Minimum of one year's experience in a supervisory role within the health/fitness or aquatics industry
- Minimum of three year's experience as a lifeguard or WSI instructor preferred

Education:

- College certificate or associate's degree in exercise science, aquatics, health, kinesiology, or recreation; bachelor's or higher degree preferred

Certification/License:

- Current YMCA, Red Cross, or other nationally recognized aquatics certification, certification as an aquatics facility operator, and/or water safety instructor
- Certified pool operator (CPO)
- Advanced life-saving and/or Red Cross lifeguard certification
- AED/CPR certification

*Adapted from Stephen J. Tharrett and James A. Peterson. *Fitness Management (2nd Edition).* Monterey, CA: Healthy Learning; 2008.

A-5g Position Title: Aquatics Staff (Lifeguard)

Position Summary:

The position of lifeguard exists to provide users and guests with a safe and enjoyable aquatics environment.

Essential Accountabilities & Functions:

- To provide a clean, well-maintained, and safe aquatics environment in compliance with both facility and local public health department standards
- To provide users with a safe and enjoyable experience within the context of the aquatics environment
- To help connect users to other users through ongoing contact with the users and the promotion of facility activities

Specific Job Accountabilities:

- Provide a welcoming greeting to users/guests when they enter the aquatics area.
- Monitor user activity within the aquatics environment to ensure a safe aquatics environment at all times.
- Assists supervisor with monitoring the pool environment to ensure that it meets all required local health codes and user needs, a responsibility that may include monitoring and balancing water chemistry, monitoring and maintaining pool temperature, and monitoring and maintaining the cleanliness of the pool.
- Assist with the maintenance of a clean and safe pool environment through proper cleaning and preventative maintenance of aquatics equipment, filter room equipment, heaters, and pool surfaces per organizational policy/procedures.
- Administer aquatics services, as set forth by the facility, including teaching swim lessons, supervising group-swim activities, and helping with other aquatics program activities.
- Assist with any required job activity of the department, as may be needed, so as to ensure users are always served in accordance with the facility's overall service philosophy.
- Behave at all times in a manner of professionalism that aligns with the values, philosophies, and standards of the facility.
- Attend all scheduled employee meetings.
- Perform other facility -related duties, as may be needed to ensure the satisfaction and enjoyment of the users.

*Adapted from Stephen J. Tharrett and James A. Peterson. *Fitness Management (2nd Edition).* Monterey, CA Healthy Learning; 2008.

Reporting Relationships:

- Reports to: Aquatics director/supervisor
- Directly supervises: N/A
- Indirectly supervises: N/A

Work Experience:

- Minimum of three month's work experience as a lifeguard preferred

Education:

- High school diploma or equivalent preferred, but not required

Certification/License:

- Certification in life saving and/or water safety from the American Red Cross or other recognized agency
- Certification in AED/CPR

*Adapted from Stephen J. Tharrett and James A. Peterson. *Fitness Management (2nd Edition).* Monterey, CA: Healthy Learning; 2008.

A-5h Position Title: Group-Exercise Coordinator/Director

Position Summary:

The group-exercise coordinator is responsible for supervising the facility's group-exercise program, including leading and instructing the various group-exercise classes offered to the users and guests of the facility.

Essential Accountabilities & Functions:

- To ensure that the facility offers a dynamic, state-of-the-art group-exercise program that attracts high user participation
- To select, develop, and supervise the group-exercise staff, with input from facility management
- To ensure that classes are well received by the user of the facility
- To ensure that each user and guest who enters the group-exercise studio is greeted with a positive attitude and that group-exercise instructors get to know each individual by name.
- To provide users with an entertaining, effective, and safe group-exercise experience whenever they participate in a class
- To provide support in properly maintaining the group-exercise studio

Specific Job Accountabilities:

- Oversee the development of the facility's group-exercise program, including developing the class schedule and format, monitoring class attendance, and recommending programs that will enhance the overall experience of individuals in the group-exercise program.
- Recruit, develop, and supervise the group-exercise staff, including overseeing all new instructor orientations, performing regular (e.g., annual) performance assessments, and making sure all classes have an instructor.
- Greet each user and guest by name when they enter and leave the group-exercise classroom.
- Come to the class at least 10 minutes in advance, prepared to provide an entertaining, effective, and safe group-exercise program for the participants.
- Promote the facility's services to users and guests.
- Assist in facilitating personal contact between users when they are in the classroom.
- Assist with the organization and preventative maintenance of the group-exercise equipment and the classroom.
- Willingly step in and assist with other facility service responsibilities, as may be required to ensure that the facility delivers upon its MFA commitment to excellence.

*Adapted from Stephen J. Tharrett and James A. Peterson. *Fitness Management (2nd Edition)*. Monterey, CA: Healthy Learning; 2008.

Reporting Relationships:

- Reports to: Fitness supervisor/director and/or facility director/general manager
- Indirectly reports to: Facility director/general manager

Work Experience:

- Minimum of three year's experience as a group-exercise instructor preferred
- Minimum of one year's experience in developing or overseeing a group-exercise program
- Teaching experience, which should include classes similar to those to be instructed at the facility

Education:

- College certificate or associate's degree in fitness/exercise science or related field; bachelor's degree preferred

Certification/License:

- Current NCCA-accredited certification as a group-exercise instructor or leader
- If instructing classes in yoga, Pilates, spinning, or related specialty class, must have either a nationally recognized certification in that specialty area or evidence of training in that specialty area
- AED/CPR certification

*Adapted from Stephen J. Tharrett and James A. Peterson. *Fitness Management (2nd Edition).* Monterey, CA: Healthy Learning; 2008.

A-5i Position Title: Group-Exercise Instructor

Position Summary:

The group-fitness instructor is responsible for leading and instructing the various group-exercise classes offered to the users and guests of the facility.

Essential Accountabilities & Functions:

- To greet each user and guest who enters the group-exercise area with an enthusiastic attitude and ensure that they get to know that individual by name
- To provide users with an entertaining, effective, and safe group-exercise experience whenever they participate in a class
- To provide support in properly maintaining the group-exercise classroom

Specific Job Accountabilities:

- Greet each user and guest by name when they enter and leave the group-exercise classroom.
- Come to the class at least 10 minutes in advance, prepared to provide an entertaining, effective, and safe group-exercise program for the participants.
- Promote the facility's services to users and guests.
- Assist in facilitating personal contact between users when they are in the classroom.
- Assist with the organization and preventative maintenance of the group-exercise equipment and studio.
- Willingly step in and assist with other facility service responsibilities, as may be required to ensure that the facility delivers upon its MFA commitment to excellence.

Reporting Relationships:

- Reports to: Group-exercise coordinator/director
- Indirectly reports to: Fitness supervisor/director

Work Experience:

- Minimum of one year's experience or 200 hours as a group-exercise instructor preferred.
- Teaching experience must include classes similar to those to be instructed at the facility.

*Adapted from Stephen J. Tharrett and James A. Peterson. *Fitness Management (2nd Edition).* Monterey, CA: Healthy Learning; 2008.

Education:

- Minimum of a high school education, with an undergraduate degree in fitness, kinesiology, or a related field preferred

Certification/License:

- Current NCCA-accredited certification as a group-exercise instructor or leader
- If instructing classes in yoga, Pilates, spinning, or related specialty class, must have either a nationally recognized certification in that specialty or evidence of training in that specialty
- AED/CPR certification

*Adapted from Stephen J. Tharrett and James A. Peterson. *Fitness Management (2nd Edition).* Monterey, CA: Healthy Learning; 2008.

A-5j Position Title: Front-Desk Receptionist

Position Summary:

The front-desk receptionist is responsible for insuring that users and guests receive a warm welcome each time they visit or call the facility. In addition, this individual is responsible for making sure that only authorized users and guests are allowed access to the facility.

Essential Accountabilities & Functions:

- To greet each user and guest with a positive attitude when they enter and leave the facility and make sure their first and last impressions of the facility are very positive
- To answer all incoming phone calls to the facility with an upbeat service attitude and to make sure that the calls are handled in a manner that addresses the needs of the caller
- To provide friendly service support in addressing the needs of the users and guests, including scheduling appointments, taking messages, answering questions from users and guests, etc.

Specific Job Accountabilities:

- Greet each user and guest by name when they enter and depart the facility.
- Check-in all users and guests when they arrive, including recording their attendance via the facility's approved systems.
- Answer the phones and handle each call so that the caller's needs are addressed.
- Perform basic operational responsibilities, such as scheduling appointments for personal training, cleaning, folding, and distributing towels, answering general questions from users and guests, handing out headphones and locks, etc.
- Appropriately process all point-of-sale transactions and member payments, according to facility policy and procedures.
- Oversee/maintain the cleanliness of the reception area of the facility.
- Willingly step in and assist with other facility service responsibilities as may be required to insure that the facility delivers upon its MFA commitment to excellence.

Reporting Relationships:

- Reports to: Member services supervisor/manager or facility director/general manager
- Indirectly reports to: N/A

*Adapted from Stephen J. Tharrett and James A. Peterson. *Fitness Management (2nd Edition).* Monterey, CA: Healthy Learning; 2008.

Work Experience:

- Minimum of one year's experience as a receptionist or similar position involving greeting customers and answering phones
- Previous work experience answering phones desirable
- Previous experience with computers, particularly with Microsoft® Office applications, desirable
- Previous experience with cash and credit card transactions/point-of-sale

Education:

- Minimum of a high school education, with some undergraduate education desirable

Certification/License:

- AED/CPR certification

*Adapted from Stephen J. Tharrett and James A. Peterson. *Fitness Management (2nd Edition).* Monterey, CA: Healthy Learning; 2008.

A-5k Position Title: Supervisor on Duty (SOD)

Position Summary:

The SOD has primary responsibility within the facility for handling emergencies, maintenance, safety, and security. The SOD serves as the first-responder to all incidents and accidents. The SOD is also responsible for ensuring that all access points to the facility are secured at the appropriate times, identifying and attending to maintenance issues, and checking up on basic safety factors (e.g., that no fire hazards exist.

Essential Accountabilities & Functions:

- To serve as the first-responder to all incidents and accidents
- To provide as much first aid as is appropriate to the level of training the SOD possesses
- To administer or oversee the administration of CPR and AED intervention, as needed
- To conduct a walk-through routine upon the start of the daily shift
- To periodically walk-through the facility during the shift, checking for maintenance, hazardous conditions, and safety factors that need attention.
- To write-out a work order for all maintenance issues unless they require immediate attention
- To undertake a closing walk-through routine that includes performing security-related closing duties

Specific Job Accountabilities:

- Oversee the execution of the facility's emergency-response plan.
- Serve as a point-of-contact for issues that arise during the shift involving maintenance, security, and safety.
- Monitor the various areas of the facility, as needed.
- Be engaged in the facility's procedures for accounting for and securing cash on hand in the facility at the end of the day.
- Oversee the efforts to ensure that the facility is secure, that no undue hazards or safety issues exist within the facility, and that all equipment is properly maintained.
- Make sure that the facility is properly secured before closing.

Reporting Relationships:

- Reports to: General manager
- Indirectly reports to: All department heads
- Directly supervises: Frontline staff
- Indirectly supervises: N/A

Education:

- College certificate or associate's degree in exercise science, health/wellness, fitness, recreation, or a related field; bachelor's degree preferred

Certification/License:

- Certification from a NCCA-accredited fitness organization, such as ACSM, ACE, NSCA, NASM, etc.
- Certification in AED/CPR

Appendix A-6
Sample Centers for Medicare & Medicaid Services Guideline

20.10—Cardiac Rehabilitation Programs (Effective March 22, 2006)

(Rev. 52, Issued: 04-21-06, Effective: 03-22-06, Implementation: 06-21-06) CIM 35-25

A. General

Phase II cardiac rehabilitation, as described by the U.S. Public Health Service, is a comprehensive, long-term program including medical evaluation, prescribed exercise, cardiac risk factor modification, education, and counseling. Phase II refers to outpatient, medically supervised programs that are typically initiated 1-3 weeks after hospital discharge and provide appropriate electrocardiographic monitoring.

B. Nationally Covered Indications

Effective for services performed on or after March 22, 2006, Medicare coverage of cardiac rehabilitation programs is considered reasonable and necessary only for patients who: (1) have a documented diagnosis of acute myocardial infarction within the preceding 12 months; or (2) have had coronary bypass surgery; or (3) have stable angina pectoris; or (4) have had heart valve repair/replacement; or (5) have had percutaneous transluminal coronary angioplasty (PTCA) or coronary stenting; or (6) have had a heart or heart-lung transplant.

1. *Program Requirements:*

a. Duration

Services provided in connection with a cardiac rehabilitation exercise program may be considered reasonable and necessary for up to 36 sessions. Patients generally receive 2 to 3 sessions per week for 12 to 18 weeks. Coverage of additional sessions is discussed in section D below.

b. Components

Cardiac rehabilitation programs must be comprehensive and to be comprehensive they must include a medical evaluation, a program to modify cardiac risk factors (e.g., nutritional counseling), prescribed exercise, education, and counseling.

c. Facility

The facility must have available for immediate use the necessary cardio-pulmonary, emergency, diagnostic, and therapeutic life-saving equipment accepted by the medical community as medically necessary, e.g., oxygen, cardiopulmonary resuscitation equipment, or defibrillator.

d. Staff

The program must be staffed by personnel necessary to conduct the program safely and effectively, who are trained in both basic and advanced life support techniques and in exercise therapy for coronary disease. The program must be under the direct supervision of a physician, as defined in 42 CFR §410.26(a)(2) (defined through cross reference to 42 CFR §410.32(b)(3)(ii), or 42 CFR §410.27(f)).

C. Nationally Non-Covered Indications

Except as provided in section D., all other indications are not covered.

D. Other

The contractor has the discretion to cover cardiac rehabilitation services beyond 18 weeks. Coverage must not exceed a total of 72 sessions for 36 weeks.

(This NCD last reviewed March 2006.)

*For additional information on other Centers for Medicare & Medicaid Services regulations, codes, and guidelines, visit www.cms.hhs.gov/home/reqsguidance.asp.

Appendix A-7
101 Reasons to Exercise

By Cedric X. Bryant, Ph.D., FACSM and James A. Peterson, Ph.D., FACSM

Research overwhelmingly shows that regular exercise lowers the risk for many diseases, enhances the functioning of virtually every physiological system in the human body and improves psychological well-being. Unfortunately, fewer than 40 percent of Americans exercise enough to experience significant health benefits. As the following list indicates, 101 extraordinarily positive reasons exist for you to exercise on a regular basis. It is well-documented that exercise:

1. Helps you to more effectively manage stress.
2. Helps you to lose weight—especially fat weight.
3. Improves the functioning of your immune system.
4. Reduces medical and healthcare expenses.
5. Reduces your risk of getting heart disease.
6. Increases your level of muscle strength.
7. Improves athletic performance.
8. Can help relieve the pain of tension headaches—perhaps the most common type of headache.
9. Allows you to consume greater quantities of food and still maintain caloric balance.
10. Helps you sleep easier and better.
11. Enhances sexual desire, performance, and satisfaction.
12. Reduces the risk of developing hypertension (high blood pressure).
13. Increases the density and breaking strength of bones.
14. Improves your physical appearance.
15. Increases circulating levels of HDL (good) cholesterol.
16. Assists in efforts to stop smoking.
17. Helps you to relax.
18. Can help improve short-term memory in older individuals.
19. Helps to maintain weight loss—unlike just dieting.
20. Helps relieve many of the common discomforts of pregnancy (backache, heartburn, constipation, etc.).
21. Reduces your anxiety level.
22. Helps control blood pressure in people with hypertension.

23. Protects against "creeping obesity" (the slow, but steady, weight gain that occurs as you age).
24. Reduces vulnerability to various cardiac dysrhythmias (abnormal heart rhythms).
25. Improves the likelihood of survival from a myocardial infarction (heart attack).
26. Helps to overcome jet lag.
27. Slows the rate of joint degeneration in people with osteoarthritis.
28. Lowers your resting heart rate.
29. Helps to boost creativity.
30. Reduces circulating levels of triglycerides.
31. Helps you resist upper-respiratory tract infections.
32. Increases your anaerobic threshold, allowing you to work or exercise longer at a higher level, before a significant amount of lactic acid builds up.
33. Helps to preserve lean body tissue.
34. Improves your ability to recover from physical exertion.
35. Helps speed recovery from chemotherapy treatments.
36. Increases ability to supply blood to the skin for cooling.
37. Increases the thickness of the cartilage in your joints.
38. Gives you more energy to meet the demands of daily life, and provides you with a reserve to meet the demands of unexpected emergencies.
39. Increases your level of muscle endurance.
40. Helps prevent intestinal ulcers.
41. Increases the density and breaking strength of ligaments and tendons.
42. Improves posture.
43. Increases your maximal oxygen uptake ($\dot{V}O_2$ max—perhaps the best measure of your physical working capacity).
44. Helps you to maintain your resting metabolic rate.
45. Reduces the risk of developing colon cancer.
46. Increases your tissues' responsiveness to the actions of insulin (i.e., improves tissue sensitivity for insulin), which helps to better control blood sugar, particularly if you are a type 2 diabetic.
47. Helps to relieve constipation.
48. Expands blood plasma volume.
49. Reduces the risk of developing prostate cancer.
50. Helps to combat substance abuse.
51. Helps to alleviate depression.
52. Increases your ability to adapt to cold environments.
53. Helps you maintain proper muscle balance.
54. Reduces the rate and severity of medical complications associated with hypertension.
55. Helps to alleviate certain menstrual symptoms.
56. Lowers your heart-rate response to submaximal physical exertion.
57. Helps to alleviate low-back pain.
58. Helps to reduce the amount of insulin required to control blood-sugar levels in type 1 (insulin-dependent) diabetics.
59. Improves mental alertness.

60. Improves respiratory muscle strength and muscle endurance—particularly important for asthmatics.
61. Reduces your risk of having a stroke.
62. Helps you to burn excess calories.
63. Increases your cardiac reserve.
64. Improves coronary (heart) circulation.
65. Offsets some of the negative side effects of certain antihypertensive drugs.
66. Increases your stroke volume (the amount of blood the heart pumps with each beat).
67. Improves your self-esteem.
68. Reduces your susceptibility for coronary thrombosis (a clot in an artery that supplies the heart with blood).
69. Reduces your risk of developing type 2 (non-insulin-dependent) diabetes.
70. Reduces the risk of developing breast cancer.
71. Improves mental cognition (a short-term effect only).
72. Maintains or improves joint flexibility.
73. Improves your glucose tolerance.
74. Reduces workdays missed due to illness.
75. Reduces the viscosity of your blood.
76. Enhances your muscles' ability to extract oxygen from your blood.
77. Increases your productivity at work.
78. Reduces your likelihood of developing low-back problems.
79. Improves your balance and coordination.
80. Improves your body's ability to use fat for energy during physical activity.
81. Provides protection against injury.
82. Decreases (by 20 to 30 percent) the need for antihypertensive medication, if you are hypertensive.
83. Improves your decision-making abilities.
84. Helps reduce and prevent the immediate symptoms of menopause (hot flashes, sleep disturbances, irritability) and decrease the long-term risks of cardiovascular disease, osteoporosis, and obesity.
85. Helps to relieve and prevent migraine-headache attacks.
86. Reduces the risk of endometriosis (a common cause of infertility).
87. Helps to retard bone loss as you age, thereby reducing your risk of developing osteoporosis.
88. Helps decrease your appetite (a short-term effect only).
89. Improves pain tolerance and mood if you suffer from osteoarthritis.
90. Helps prevent and relieve the stresses that cause carpal tunnel syndrome.
91. Makes your heart a more efficient pump.
92. Helps to decrease left ventricular hypertrophy (a thickening of the walls of the left ventricle) in people with hypertension.
93. May be protective against the development of Alzheimer's disease.
94. Improves your mood.
95. Helps to increase your overall health awareness.
96. Reduces the risk of gastrointestinal bleeding.
97. Helps you to maintain an independent lifestyle.
98. Reduces the level of abdominal obesity—a significant health-risk factor.

99. Increases the diffusion capacity of the lungs, enhancing the exchange of oxygen from your lungs to your blood.
100. Improves heat tolerance.
101. Improves your overall quality of life.

A Wise Investment Strategy

According to the Centers for Disease Control and Prevention, if the millions of sedentary Americans started exercising regularly, they would save billions annually in medical costs. On average, each inactive American spends approximately $330 more per year on healthcare expenses than their active counterparts. The evidence is conclusive: exercise is a wise investment. It offers countless health benefits at virtually no cost. Over time, as you sustain your commitment to being physically active, not only will you reap the financial rewards, you'll also be more physically and emotionally able to enjoy the fruits of your investment.

Appendix B Forms

B-1. Sample Pre-Activity Screening Forms
- Pre-Activity Screening Form
- Cardiovascular Health Pre-Activity Screening Form
- Health History Inventory Form
- Physical Fitness Profile Form

B-2. Sample Risk-Management Forms
- Authorization for Release of Protected Health Information Form
- Emergency Medical Authorization Form
- Activity Release and Indemnity Agreement—Adult Form
- Waiver and Release—Adult Form
- AED Site Survey Worksheet
- AED Program Implementation Checklist
- AED Maintenance Checklist
- Incident Report Form

B-3. Sample Area-Specific Usage Guidelines and Policies
- Cardiovascular Area Usage Guidelines and Policies
- Strength Fitness Area Usage Guidelines and Policies
- Group-Exercise Studio Area Usage Guidelines and Policies
- Aquatics and Pool Area Usage Guidelines and Policies
- Locker Room Usage Guidelines and Policies

B-4. Sample Professional Staffing Forms
- Employee Development Plan Form
- Employee Performance Objectives—Semi-Annual Form
- New Employee Orientation Checklist
- Compensation Agreement (Salaried Employee)
- Compensation Agreement (Hourly and/or Commission Employee)

B-5. Sample Operational Policies and Procedures Forms
- Equipment Maintenance Log Sheet
- Maintenance and Repair Service Request Form
- Opening Report Form

B-6. Sample Quality Management Forms
- Strategic Planning Worksheet
- Strategic Plan Action Worksheet
- Program Best Practices Benchmark Form
- User Feedback Form

Appendix B-1
Sample Pre-Activity Screening Forms

- Pre-Activity Screening Form
- Cardiovascular Health Pre-Activity Screening Form
- Health History Inventory Form
- Physical Fitness Profile Form

B-1a. Pre-Activity Screening Form

(Name of Center)
Pre-Activity Screening

Name: ____________________ Member/Client Number: ____________________

Address: ____

Telephone (W): ____________________ Telephone (H): ____________________

Fax: ____________________ E-mail: ____________________

Gender: ____________________ Birth date: ____________________

Regular physical activity is enjoyable, safe, and healthy for most people. However, some individuals may have health-related risks that might be aggravated by participation in a physical-activity program, and, as a result, might require them to check with their physician prior to embarking on a physical-activity program. To help determine if there is a need for you to see your physician before beginning an exercise program, please answer the following questions carefully. All information will be kept strictly confidential.

I. PRE-ACTIVITY SCREENING QUESTIONS

Yes	No	
❑	❑	1. Has your physician ever told you that you have a heart condition?
❑	❑	2. Do you experience pain in your chest when you are physically active?
❑	❑	3. In the past month, have you experienced chest pain when not performing physical activity?
❑	❑	4. Do you lose balance because of dizziness or do you ever lose consciousness?
❑	❑	5. Do you have a bone or joint problem that could be aggravated by a change in your level of physical activity?
❑	❑	6. Is your physician currently prescribing medications for your blood pressure or a heart condition?
❑	❑	7. Do you know of any other reason why you should not participate in a physical-activity program?

If you answered yes to any of the questions above, it is recommended that you consult with your physician, by phone or in person, before having a fitness test or participating in a physical-activity program.

B-1b. Cardiovascular Health Pre-Activity Screening Form

(Name of Center)

Cardiovascular Health Pre-Activity Screening

For each of the following questions, please place a check mark by each item that directly applies to you.

1. ❑ Age: Men >45 Women >55
2. ❑ Family history: myocardial infarction or sudden death before 55 years of age for father, other first-degree male relative, or 65 years of age for mother or female first-degree relative
3. ❑ Cigarette smoker: (Current or quit in the past six months)
4. ❑ Hypercholesterolemia:

   Total cholesterol >200 mg/dL

   LDL cholesterol >130 mg/dL

   HDL <40 mg/dL
5. ❑ Hypertension: Blood pressure—Systolic BP greater than or equal to 140 mmHg or diastolic BP greater than or equal to 90 mmHg, or on antihypertensive medications
6. ❑ Impaired fasting glucose: Fasting blood glucose greater than or equal to 100 mg/dL
7. ❑ Obesity: Body Mass Index >30 or waist circumference >40 (men) and >35 (women)
8. ❑ Sedentary lifestyle: Not meeting the minimum physical activity guidelines of the U.S. Surgeon General's Report (30 minutes of moderate physical activity most days of the week)

Place a check in the line below that applies to the member.

❑ Apparently healthy:

Individuals who are asymptomatic and apparently healthy with no more than one major coronary risk factor

Risk factors: ______________________________

____

❑ Moderate risk:

Individuals who have signs or symptoms of possible cardiopulmonary or metabolic disease and/or two or more major coronary risk factors. Physician's note needed.

Risk factors: ______________________________

____

❑ High risk/known disease.

Individuals with known cardiac, pulmonary, or metabolic disease. Physician's note needed.

Risk factors: ______________________________

____

B-1c. Health History Inventory Form

(Name of Center)

Health History Inventory (Long version)

Please answer each of the questions in this inventory to the best of your ability. For each question, please mark the best choice, unless otherwise indicated. In some instances, you will need to write out your response. If you need assistance with answering any of these questions, please request assistance from a fitness professional. All of your responses will be treated in a confidential manner.

GENERAL INFORMATION

Name: ______________________________

Gender: ❑ Male ❑ Female Birth Date: ______________________

Height: _____ ft. _____ inches Weight: ____________ pounds

Address: ______________________________

City: ______________________ State: _________ ZIP: __________

Phone (office): ________________ Phone (cell): ________________

Phone (home): ________________ E-mail: ________________

Marital Status: ________________ Highest Level of Education Attained: __________

Occupation: ______________________________

Primary Care Physician: ______________________________

Address: ______________________________

City: ______________________ State: _________ ZIP: __________

Phone (office): ________________

Program Goals (i.e., your training objectives): ______________________________

PART I: PAST MEDICAL HISTORY

1. Have you ever been told by a doctor that you have or had heart problems, an abnormal EKG, or had a heart attack or stroke? ❑ Yes ❑ No
2. Have you ever had coronary by-pass surgery, angioplasty, or any other type of heart surgery? ❑ Yes ❑ No
3. Have you ever had difficulty breathing or become short of breath with mild or light exertion? ❑ Yes ❑ No
4. Do you have a history of diabetes or thyroid, kidney, or liver disease? ❑ Yes ❑ No
5. Have you ever experienced irregular heartbeat (arrhythmia) or been diagnosed with a heart condition or disease? ❑ Yes ❑ No
6. If you answered YES to any of the above questions, please provide additional information below:

____

____

B-1c. Health History Inventory Form *continued*

PART II: CURRENT MEDICAL HISTORY

7. Do you currently experience or have any of the following:
   a. Pain or discomfort in the chest or surrounding areas that occurs when you engage in exercise or physical activity? ❑ Yes ❑ No
   b. Shortness of breath with activity or at rest? ❑ Yes ❑ No
   c. Unexplained dizziness or fainting? ❑ Yes ❑ No
   d. Difficulty breathing at night, except in an upright position? ❑ Yes ❑ No
   e. Swelling in the ankles or lower extremities (other than due to an injury)? ❑ Yes ❑ No
   f. Heart palpitations (rapid or irregular heart beat of the heart)? ❑ Yes ❑ No
   g. Pain in the legs that may cause you to stop walking? ❑ Yes ❑ No
   h. Known heart murmur? ❑ Yes ❑ No
8. Are you pregnant or is it likely that you may become pregnant at this time? ❑ Yes ❑ No
   If you are pregnant, what is your expected due date? ______________________
9. Have you had surgery, or been diagnosed with any disease in the past three months? ❑ Yes ❑ No
   If you answered yes to question 9, please list the date ______________________
   And nature of the surgery/disease: ______________________
10. In the past 12 months, have you been told by a healthcare professional that you have an elevated cholesterol level or abnormal lipid profile, or are you on any medications to control your blood lipids? ❑ Yes ❑ No
11. Do you currently smoke cigarettes, or have you quit within the past six months? ❑ Yes ❑ No
12. Have your father or brother(s) had heart disease prior to the age of 55 or mother or sister(s) had heart disease prior to age 65? ❑ Yes ❑ No
13. Within the past 12 months, has a healthcare professional told you that you have high blood pressure? (systolic >140 mmHg, diastolic >90 mmHg) ❑ Yes ❑ No
14. Do you currently have high blood pressure, or are you taking medication(s) to manage high blood pressure? ❑ Yes ❑ No
15. Within the past 12 months, have you been told by a healthcare professional that you have an elevated fasting blood glucose level? (>100 mg/dl) ❑ Yes ❑ No
16. Are you currently under the care of a healthcare professional for blood clots or other circulatory problems? ❑ Yes ❑ No
17. Do you currently experience problems or pain in your bones, joints, or muscles that may be aggravated with exercise? ❑ Yes ❑ No
18. Do you currently experience any back and/or neck discomfort or problems? ❑ Yes ❑ No
19. Are you currently under the care of a healthcare professional for any other health/medical problems? ❑ Yes ❑ No

B-1c. Health History Inventory Form *continued*

20. If you have answered YES to any of the questions in part II (questions 7–19), please provide additional information below:

____

____

21. Please list below all prescription and over-the-counter medications you are currently taking?

Medicine	Dosage	Frequency

22. Are there any medications that your physician and/or healthcare professional have prescribed for you in the past 12 months that you are currently not taking? ❑ Yes ❑ No

    If you answered yes, please list the medications? ____________________

PART III: PHYSICAL ACTIVITY/EXERCISE HISTORY

23. Please list any favorite activities you would like to include in your exercise plan.

____

____

24. Please list any activities you dislike or do not want to include in your exercise plan.

____

____

25. Please list any fitness activities (e.g., jogging, cycling, strength training) that you participate in regularly (include how often, how hard, and how long).

____

____

26. Please list any recreational activities (e.g., golf, tennis) that you participate in regularly (include how often).

____

____

27. Where do you plan to exercise (e.g., club, home, outdoors)?

____

____

28. If you plan to exercise at home, list all available equipment.

____

____

29. Have you been told by a healthcare professional that you should not exercise? ❑ Yes ❑ No

B-1c. Health History Inventory Form *continued*

30. If you answered YES to question #29 in part III, please describe below:

____

____

____

PART IV: WEIGHT HISTORY

31. What do you consider to be your ideal body weight? __________
32. What has been your lowest body weight as an adult (list how old you were)? __________
33. What has been your highest body weight as an adult (list how old you were)? __________
34. What is your current weight? __________
35. What was your weight one year ago? __________

PART V: DIET/NUTRITION HISTORY

36. How many meals do you typically eat per day? __________
37. Do you eat a variety of foods from each of the food groups? ❑ Yes ❑ No
38. Do you try to limit the amount of fat you eat to <30% of your total daily caloric intake? ❑ Yes ❑ No
39. Do you use sugar sparingly by adding little or none to the foods you eat and by limiting your intake of desserts, candy, and soft drinks? ❑ Yes ❑ No
40. Do you limit your alcohol consumption to 1–2 drinks or fewer per day? ❑ Yes ❑ No
41. If you answered NO to any of the questions in part V (questions 37–40), please describe below:

____

____

____

I have answered the questions in this Health History Inventory to the best of my ability, and as accurately and completely as possible. I understand that this information is kept strictly confidential and is used only for the purpose of helping the health/fitness professional make the most appropriate recommendations and design a safe and effective physical-activity program to meet my unique needs. Furthermore, I understand that this information cannot be released to any other party without my prior written approval in accordance with the Health Insurance Portability and Accountability Act of 1996. I understand that my failure to disclose health, medical, or related information that might affect my participation in physical activity may limit the ability of the health/fitness professional to provide the safest possible physical-activity program. Finally, I understand that the information collected in this Health History Inventory has been designed using the recommendations provided by the American College of Sports Medicine for risk stratification as described in the publication, *ACSM's Guidelines for Exercise Testing and Prescription, 7th edition (2006).*

Client/member signature: ____________________ Date: __________

Staff/trainer signature: ____________________ Date: __________

B-1c. Health History Inventory Form *continued*

For Use by a Qualified Fitness Professional—Health History Inventory II

1. Check off the major coronary risk factors as described by the American College of Sports Medicine in their publication, *ACSM's Guidelines for Exercise Testing and Prescription, 7th edition (2006).*
   - ❑ Dyslipidemia (total cholesterol over 200 mg/dL, LDL over 130 mg/dL, HDL less than 40 mg/dL, or on lipid medication)
   - ❑ Hypertension (systolic BP >140 mmHg, diastolic BP >90 mmHg as confirmed by two measurements)
   - ❑ Cigarette smoking (current smoker or stopped within the past 6 months)
   - ❑ Impaired fasting glucose (fasting level >100 mg/dL)
   - ❑ Obesity (body mass index >30; waist/hip ratio greater than 0.95 for men and 0.86 for women)
   - ❑ Sedentary lifestyle (person does not participate in a regular exercise program)
   - ❑ Family history (history of heart attack or heart surgery before age 55 on the male side of the family and before age 65 on the female side of the family)
2. Risk Stratification
   - ❑ Low Risk (men < age 45 or women < age 55 who are asymptomatic and have no more than one risk factor)

     No physician clearance required for this person to engage in a program of moderate physical activity.
   - ❑ Moderate Risk (men > age 45 and women > age 55, or those who have two or more risk factors at any age)

     Physician/medical clearance required before this person can engage in a program of moderate physical activity.
   - ❑ High Risk (individuals having one or more signs or symptoms, or having known cardiovascular, pulmonary, or metabolic disease)

     Physician/medical clearance required before this person can engage in a program of moderate physical activity.

Additional Comments:

____

____

____

____

____

____

____

____

B-1d. Physical Fitness Profile Form

Date of Profile Administration: ______________________________
Client/Member Name: ______________________________
Birth Date: ______________ Gender: ❑ Male ❑ Female
Height: ______ feet ______ inches ______ meters Weight: ______ pounds ______ kilograms
Supine Resting HR: ______ Seated/Standing RHR: ______
Supine Resting BP: ______ Seated/Standing RBP: ______

CARDIOVASCULAR ASSESSMENT PROFILE

Estimated Maximum HR: ________ Estimated 85% of Maximum HR: ________

Rockport Walk Test:	______ min	______ sec		HR: ______		RPE: ______
3-Minute Step Test:	______ min	______ sec		HR: ______		RPE: ______
YMCA Bike Test	Stage 1	______ HR	______ KPM			RPE: ______
	Stage 2	______ HR	______ KPM			RPE: ______
	Stage 3	______ HR	______ KPM			RPE: ______
	Stage 4	______ HR	______ KPM			RPE: ______

Estimated Maximum $\dot{V}O_2$ (mL/kg/min): ________

BODY COMPOSITION PROFILE

a. Girth Measurements

Arm	______ inches	______ cm
Chest	______ inches	______ cm
Umbilical	______ inches	______ cm
Hips	______ inches	______ cm
Thigh	______ inches	______ cm
Calf	______ inches	______ cm

Waist/hip ratio: ________
Estimated % Bodyfat: ________

b. Skinfold Measurements

Pectoral	______ mm
Tricep	______ mm
Scapula	______ mm
Axilla	______ mm
Abdomen	______ mm
Illium	______ mm
Thigh	______ mm
Sum Skinfolds	______ mm

MUSCULAR STRENGTH AND ENDURANCE PROFILE

a. Muscular Strength

Bench Press (1 RM) ______ lbs
Leg Press (1 RM) ______ lbs

b. Muscular Endurance

Push-ups ______ reps
Curl-up ______ reps
YMCA Bench ______ reps

FLEXIBILITY PROFILE

a. Shoulder Girdle

Flexion ______ degrees
Extension ______ degrees
Horizontal Abduction ______ degrees
Horizontal Adduction ______ degrees

b. Trunk/Core

Flexion ______ degrees
Extension ______ degrees
Lateral Flexion ______ degrees
Rotation ______ degrees

c. Hips

Flexion ______ degrees
Extension ______ degrees
Abduction ______ degrees
Adduction ______ degrees

The benchmarks and protocols for each of the assessment measurements on this form are based on the recommendations of the American College of Sports Medicine as highlighted in the publication, *ACSM's Guidelines for Exercise Testing and Prescription, 7th edition (2006).*

Appendix B-2
Selected Risk-Management Forms*

- Authorization for Release of Protected Health Information Form
- Emergency Medical Authorization Form
- Activity Release and Indemnity Agreement—Adult Form
- Waiver and Release—Adult Form
- AED Site Survey Worksheet
- AED Program Implementation Checklist
- AED Maintenance Checklist
- Incident Report Form

*Because the selected risk management forms in this appendix can represent a form of legal document, before using them, corporate risk manager and/or legal counsel should review them concerning their application to state and local laws, which can vary from location to location.

B-2a. Authorization for Release of Protected Health Information Form

(Name of Center)

Authorization for Release of Protected Health Information

I, ______________________________ , hereby authorize ______________________________ to release the following health information:

and forward it to the following person/facility:

Name or person or facility: ______________________________

Address (street, city, state and zip code):

Phone #: ______________________ Email: ______________________________

This information is for the purpose of:

This authorization is in effect until ______________________________, when it expires.

I understand that by signing this authorization:

- I authorize the use or disclosure of my individually identifiable health information as described above for the purpose listed. I understand that authorization is voluntary.
- I understand the notice of Privacy Practices provides instructions should I choose to revoke my authorization.
- I understand that if the organization I have authorized to receive the information is not a health plan or health care provider, the released information may no longer be protected by federal privacy regulations.
- I understand that I have the right to receive a copy of this authorization.
- I understand that I am signing this authorization voluntarily and that treatment, payment, or eligibility for my benefits will not be affected if I do not sign this authorization.

I DECLARE UNDER PENALTY OF PERJURY THAT THE INFORMATION ON THIS FORM IS TRUE AND CORRECT.

SIGNATURE: ______________________________ **DATE:** ______________________

B-2b. Emergency Medical Authorization Form

(Name of Center)

Emergency Medical Authorization—Adult

I hereby give consent, in the event I am incapacitated and unable to provide such consent and approval for a situation requiring medical attention and action for the administration of any treatment or care deemed necessary, and my designated representative, ______________________ can not be reached in a reasonable period of time to extend such consent and approval on my behalf for attention and action for the administration of any treatment and/or care deemed necessary for the listed above by Dr. ______________________, or any of his/her associates, the preferred physician, or Dr. ______________________, or any of his/her associates, the preferred dentist, or in the event the appropriate preferred physician, dentist or other identified healthcare professional is not available, by another qualified physician, dentist or healthcare professional; and the transfer of myself to ______________________ hospital, the preferred hospital, or any hospital reasonably accessible.

This authorization does not cover non-emergency medical situations or non-emergency major surgery unless the opinions of at least two other licensed physicians, dentists or healthcare professionals concurring in the necessity of such emergency medical action are obtained prior to the performance of such emergency medical action/surgery and unless all reasonable attempts to obtain my approval and in the event I am incapable of providing such approval then efforts to contact my designated representative have been exhausted, defining such period for non-emergency medical action/surgery as 24 hours.

The following information is being released by me in the event that the physician, dentist, healthcare professional, or hospital is unable to access my medical history;

Allergies:

Medications:

Physical limitations/restrictions:

(Other critical information (e.g. blood type, health conditions, etc.):

Insurance coverage:

Insurance provider		Policy number	

B-2b. Emergency Medical Authorization Form *continued*

I the undersigned, hereby agree appoint and constitute the center, and its duly authorized representative(s), namely ______________________ , for the period of ______________________ , 20________ , through and including ______________________ , 20________ , and do hereby authorize them to obtain any x-ray examination, anesthesia, medical or surgical diagnosis or treatment, and hospital care to be provided for me in the event I am unable to provide approval and my designated representative can not be reached for approval in a reasonable period of time, under the general and special supervision, and on the advice of a licensed physician, dentist, or other qualified healthcare professional acting under their supervision.

Signature: ____

Name (print): ____

Center's representative (witness) signature: ______________________________

Center's representative name (print): ______________________________

Date: ______________________ State of ______________________

Country of ______________________

B-2c. Activity Release and Indemnity Agreement—Adult Form

(Name of Center)

Activity Release and Indemnity Agreement—Adult

THIS RELEASE AND INDEMNITY AGREEMENT ("Release") is made by the undersigned adult (the "Participant"), to release and indemnify_________________________ , a _________________________ corporation, its parent company, affiliated or subsidiary companies, and all their respective officers, directors, agents, contractors, employees, heirs, successors, and assigns (collectively, the "Center"), as set forth below.

1. **Activity.** Participant, on Participant's own behalf and on behalf of the other members of Participant's family, including Participant's spouse, parents, children, heirs, and assigns, (singularly and collectively referred to as "Participant") hereby grants to the Center this full release and indemnification as consideration in exchange for permitting Participant to participate in the following athletic or physical activity which may utilize Center premises and/or equipment (the "Activity") ____________________ .

   Participant is entering into this Release after (i) having viewed or having had the opportunity to view Center premises and/or equipment; (ii) if there is an instructor, having reviewed or having had the opportunity to review the instructor's qualifications; (iii) having had the scope of the services and/or the associated risks explained to Participant; and/or (iv) having had an opportunity to ask questions regarding the services and/or the risks associated with the Activity.

2. **Release and Indemnity.**
   - PARTICIPANT IS VOLUNTARILY PARTICIPATING IN THE ACTIVITY WITH FULL KNOWLEDGE, UNDERSTANDING AND APPRECIATION OF THE RISKS OF INJURY INHERENT IN ANY PHYSICAL EXERCISE, MASSAGE OR THERAPY PROGRAM, PHYSICAL ACTIVITY OR ATHLETIC ACTIVITY AND EXPRESSLY ASSUMES ALL RISKS OF INJURY AND EVEN DEATH WHICH COULD OCCUR BY REASON OF PARTICIPANT'S PARTICIPATION.
   - PARTICIPANT RELEASES CENTER FROM ANY LIABILITY AND AGREES NOT TO SUE CENTER WITH RESPECT TO ANY CAUSE OF ACTION FOR BODILY INJURY, PROPERTY DAMAGE, OR DEATH OCCURRING TO PARTICIPANT AS A RESULT OF PARTICIPATING IN THE ACTIVITY.
   - PARTICIPANT HEREBY ASSUMES FULL RESPONSIBILITY FOR RISKS OF BODILY INJURY, PROPERTY DAMAGE OR DEATH TO PARTICIPANT DUE TO THE ORDINARY NEGLIGENCE OR GROSS NEGLIGENCE OF THE CENTER AND THE ORDINARY NEGLIGENCE, GROSS NEGLIGENCE, OR WILLFUL MISCONDUCT OF ANY THIRD PARTY INCLUDING OTHERS PARTICIPATING IN THE ACTIVITY.
   - PARTICIPANT AGREES TO INDEMNIFY, DEFEND, AND HOLD HARMLESS, AT PARTICIPANT'S SOLE COST, THE CENTER FROM ANY AND ALL CLAIMS ARISING OUT OF PARTICIPANT'S PARTICIPATION IN THE ACTIVITY.
   - ALL PERSONAL PROPERTY BROUGHT TO THE ACTIVITY, IS BROUGHT AT THE SOLE RISK OF PARTICIPANT AS TO ITS THEFT, DAMAGE, OR LOSS.

B-2c. Activity Release and Indemnity Agreement—Adult Form *continued*

3. **Medical.** Participant consents to emergency medical care and transportation in order to obtain treatment in the event of injury to Participant as the Center may deem appropriate. This Release extends to any liability arising out of or in any way connected with the medical treatment and transportation provided in the event of an emergency.

4. **Severability.** Participant expressly agrees that the terms of release and indemnity contained herein are intended to be as broad and inclusive as is permitted by the laws of the state in which Center operates its business. Any provision or portion of this Release found to be invalid by the courts having jurisdiction shall be invalid only with respect to such provision or portion. The offending provision or portion shall be construed to the maximum extent possible to confer upon the parties the benefits intended thereby. Said provision or portion, as well as the remaining provisions or portion hereof, shall be construed and enforced to the same effect as if such offending provision or portion thereof had not been contained herein.

PARTICIPANT HAS READ AND VOLUNTARILY SIGNS THIS RELEASE AND INDEMNITY AGREEMENT.

PARTICIPANT:

____
Signature

____
Printed Name

____
Date

B-2d. Waiver and Release—Adult Form

(Name of Center)

Waiver and Release—Adult

I agree to abide by the rules of the Center, including the completion of a pre-activity screening questionnaire and/or health/medical information questionnaire prior to participation in any physical activities at the Center. I further agree that all use of the Center's facilities, programs, and services shall be undertaken at my sole risk and that the Center shall not be liable for any injuries, accidents, or death occurring to me, including those resulting from the Center's negligence, arising either directly or indirectly out of my participation in, or use of, the Center's facilities, programs, and services. I, for myself and on behalf of my executors, administrators, heirs, and assigns, do hereby expressly release, discharge, waive, relinquish, and covenant not to sue the Center, its affiliates, officers, directors, agents, or employees for all such claims, demands, injuries, damages, or causes of action, including those resulting from the Center's negligence, arising either directly or indirectly out of my participation in, or use of, the Center's facilities, programs, and services.

I declare that I have completed the Center's pre-activity screening questionnaire and/or health/medical information questionnaire and that I am physically able to participate in physical activity. Furthermore, I acknowledge that the Center has advised me to obtain a physician's clearance in the event the answers on either the pre-activity screening questionnaire and/or health/medical information questionnaire indicates that I should not participate in a program of physical activity without a physician's clearance, or if the Center is unsure of my physical health, yet I maintain that I am physically capable of pursuing physical activity in the Center without such steps being taken or has done so.

Individual's signature: ______________________________ Date: ______________

Staff witness signature: ______________________________ Date: ______________

B-2e. AED Site Survey Worksheet

AED Site Survey Worksheet	
Site Name	
Date	

Physical Location Describe building type, floors, access, grounds, parking, remote areas. Include approximate brisk walking times to key points. Attach floor plan if available.	
SCA High-Risk Areas Examples: exercise/fitness areas, high occupancy/gathering areas, swimming pools, high voltage equipment, heavy machinery.	
Response Barriers Examples: stairs, elevators, locked/secure areas, hazardous areas, crowds/congestion, roadways/ driveways.	
Population People regularly present: staff, visitors, etc. Approximate headcount. Adults? Children (<8yrs)? What hours of day? Shift workers?	
Responders Who will respond? How many? How will they be notified? Type of training. Times available to respond?	
AED Placement Location(s), quantity, time/distance to reach, accessories, oxygen, mounted/ mobile, ambient temperature, phone nearby	
Other Considerations	

Organization		**Completed by**	

B-2f. AED Program Implementation Checklist

Identify:

Program decision-makers and influencers ____

Physician to provide prescription for AED ____

Medical oversight (physician or other medical professional) ____

Targeted responders ____

State and local requirements for AEDs ____

Local EMS system requirements (if applicable) ____

Decide:

Type of AED ____

Placement of AEDs:

- Limited vs. open accessibility ____
- Secured vs. unsecured ____
- Automatic notification system: yes or no ____
- Audio-visual alarm: yes or no ____

Options on AEDs:

- Voice/environmental data: yes or no ____
- Manual override: yes or no ____
- Display screen: yes or no ____
- Modem, data card, chip or cassette tape ____

Number of AEDs ____

Method of notifying EMS ____

Method of activating internal Medical Emergency Response Plan (MERP) ____

Number of employees to be trained ____

Training program ____

Retraining program and interval:

- Skills review (refresher, update, etc.) ____
- Formal retraining ____

Method for ensuring AED readiness ____

Method for scheduling and conducting AED maintenance checks ____

Method for educating participants on how to activate the internal MERP ____

Method for internally and externally promoting the AED program and Chain of Survival for participants ____

Method for capturing data ____

Method for patient care transfer to local EMS agency ____

Method for event review ____

Methods for quality improvement ____

Method for rescuer debriefing ____

Method for putting AED back into use ____

Method for monitoring patient outcome ____

Write:

Internal response procedures for use of the AED (reflect site-specific variables such as type of AED, activation method, hazards, etc.) ____

AED maintenance procedure ____

Transfer of patient care procedure (coordinate with local EMS) ____

Contact:

State office of EMS for registration purposes (if applicable) ____

Local EMS agency ____

Local dispatch center ____

American Heart Association for training information ____

AED manufacturer if AED maintenance is needed ____

B-2g. Automated External Defibrillator Maintenance Checklist

Automated External Defibrillator Maintenance Checklist

Date		Location	

Inspection Performed by	

Criteria	Status	Corrective Action /Comments
AED		
Placement visible, unobstructed, and near phone		
Verify battery installation		
Check the status/service indicator light		
Note absence of visual/ audible service alarm		
Inspect exterior components and sockets for cracks		
Supplies		
Two sets of AED pads in sealed package		
Check expiration date on pad packages		
Pocket mask with one-way valve		
Examination gloves		
Razors		
Absorbent gauze or hand towels		

Please refer to manufacturer's user's manual for more information and proper annual maintenance procedures.

B-2h. Incident Report Form

(Name of Center)

Incident Report Form

I. General Incident Information

Month Day Year Time of Incident A.M. P.M.	Center Member ______ Yes ______ No	Center Name Center Location

	First M.I. Last	Hospital/EMS or physician notified? ______ Yes ______ No
Name of Injured Person:		Name of caller: ______
Street Address:		Time of initial call: ______
State/City/Zip:		Time of any follow-up calls: 1. ______ 2. ______ 3. ______
Phone #'s:		Time of EMS arrival: ______ Time of EMD departure: ______
Email Address:		Hospital taken to: ______ Name of EMS contact: ______

II. General Description of the Incident

Description of incident:

____

____

____

____

____

____

____

Bleeding-related injury?	______ Yes	______ No
Visible injury?	______ Yes	______ No
Not outwardly noticeable injury, but person expressed pain?	______ Yes	______ No
If an eye injury, was eyewear/protection being worn?	______ Yes	______ No

B-2h. Incident Report Form *continued*

III. Incident Details, Including Center's Response to the Incident

Description of the injury/injuries:	Description of center's response/first aid:

IV. Responder, Supervisor, and Witness Information

First responder (name):

Responders position/title;

CPR certified? ____ Yes ____ No AED certified? ____ Yes ____ No

First-aid certified? ____ Yes ____ No

Signature:

Manager on duty (name):

Manager on duty position/title:

CPR certified? ____ Yes ____ No AED certified? ____ Yes ____ No

First-aid certified? ____ Yes ____ No

Signature:

Witness (name):

Witness address: ________________________________

Witness phone: (B) ____________ (H) ____________ (C) ____________

Witness email: ____________________ Signature: ____________________

Witness (name):

Witness address: ________________________________

Witness phone: (B) ____________ (H) ____________ (C) ____________

Witness email: ____________________ Signature: ____________________

B-2h. Incident Report Form *continued*

V. Details on Location of Incident

1. Specific location:

_____ fitness center	_____ studio	_____ gymnasium
_____ pool	_____ tennis court	_____ locker rooms
_____ spa	_____ lobby/circulation area	
_____ children's	_____ steam/sauna/whirlpool (circle)	
_____ outside	_____ other	

2. Please describe the conditions of the environment during the time of the incident (e.g., was it a wet surface, was it extremely hot, etc.):

3. Other comments:

VI. Miscellaneous

1. Did the police investigate? ______ Yes ______ No If yes, please give name, rank and contact information on the lines below.

Name: ________________________ Rank: ________________________

Contact phone number: ________________________

2. Did another agency investigate (fire department, etc.) ______ Yes ______ No
If yes, please give name, rank and contact information on the lines below.

Name: ________________________ Rank: ________________________

Contact phone number: ________________________

Report submitted by: ________________________ Signature: ________________________

Date and time submitted: ________________________

Please make multiple copies, including one for the person's file, the center's incident files, the insurer, and the individual involved in the incident.

Appendix B-3
Sample Area-Specific Usage Guidelines and Policies

- Cardiovascular Fitness Area Usage Guidelines and Policies
- Strength Fitness Area Usage Guidelines and Policies
- Group-Exercise Studio Area Usage Guidelines and Policies
- Aquatics and Pool Area Usage Guidelines and Policies
- Locker Room Usage Guidelines and Policies

The forms in this section are adapted and used with permission from Stephen J. Tharrett and James A. Peterson, *Fitness Management* (2nd Edition). Monterey, CA: Healthy Learning; 2008.

B-3a. Cardiovascular Fitness Area Usage Guidelines and Policies

(Name of Center)

Cardiovascular Fitness Area Usage Guidelines and Policies

1. Engaging in any form of physical activity carries an increased risk of experiencing an event such as rapid heartbeat, dizziness, orthopedic injury, and in rare instances, stroke, sudden cardiac event, or even death. To minimize these risks, we encourage you to meet with one of the Center's fitness professionals and receive the proper screening and orientation prior to engaging in any exercise.
2. If you have any health condition that would compromise your ability to participate in exercise, please see a fitness professional before participating.
3. A target heart rate chart and chart of perceived exertion is available in the cardiovascular fitness area to assist you with monitoring the intensity of your training.
4. General guidelines for engaging in cardiovascular training are as follows:
   a. Choose a mode of activity that is comfortable and enjoyable.
   b. Activities such as walking, jogging, biking, and elliptical training are all good modes for cardiovascular training.
   c. Warm up for several minutes before actively starting your cardiovascular training.
   d. The recommended time duration for cardiovascular training is between 20 and 60 minutes of continuous or intermittent training (bouts as short as 10 minutes).
   e. The recommended intensity for cardiovascular training is between 40 and 85% of heart-rate reserve, with the recommendation for beginners being between 40 and 60%.
   f. The recommended frequency for cardiovascular conditioning is 3-to-5 times per week, with the recommendation for beginners being a minimum of two times per week.
5. The cardiovascular area is supervised by a fitness professional during all peak usage periods. During all other times, a member of the fitness staff makes regular rounds through the area.
6. In the event you need assistance, please talk to one of our fitness professionals. If one is not available, contact the front desk for assistance.
7. In the event that you witness and/or experience an event that places you or another user in harm's way, please initiate the facility's emergency response system by using the nearest phone and dialing ______________ .
8. In the event of a sudden cardiac event, the Center has an AED located at ________________________ .
9. No food and drink other than water or sports performance drinks in plastic containers are allowed in this area.
10. Please respect your fellow users by wiping down the equipment when you have finished using it.
11. During periods of peak usage, please limit yourself to a maximum of 30 minutes on any one piece of equipment. If you need to perform more than 30 minutes of exercise, please make use of other equipment so that everyone is given an equal opportunity to pursue their fitness program.
12. Cell phones must be turned off or put on vibrate.

B-3b. Strength Fitness Area Usage Guidelines and Policies

(Name of Center)

Strength Fitness Area Usage Guidelines and Policies

1. Engaging in any form of physical activity carries an increased risk of experiencing an event such as rapid heartbeat, dizziness, orthopedic injury, and in rare instances, stroke, sudden cardiac event, or even death. To minimize these risks, we encourage you to meet with one of the Center's fitness professionals and receive the proper screening and orientation prior to engaging in any exercise.

2. If you have any health condition that would compromise your ability to participate in exercise, please see a fitness professional before participating.

3. General guidelines for engaging in the resistance and/or free-weight training are as follows:
   a. Choose a mode of movement that is comfortable.
   b. Perform movements for all the major muscle groups of the body. This will normally involve 8 to 10 separate exercises that work the hips, buttocks, thighs, legs, back, chest, shoulders, arms, and abdomen.
   c. Perform 1 set of each exercise to the point of volitional fatigue. Recommendations are to perform between 3 and 20 repetitions, depending on the results you desire.
   d. Resistance and/or free-weight exercises should be performed 2 to 3 days a week, with at least one day's rest between workouts.

4. The resistance area is supervised by a fitness professional during all peak usage periods. During all other times, a member of the fitness staff makes regular rounds through the area.

5. In the event you need assistance, please talk to one of the Center's fitness professionals and if one is not available, contact the front desk for assistance.

6. We encourage the use of a spotter whenever you are performing a movement that involves exposing yourself to the possibility of a weight device falling on you.

7. In the event that you witness and/or experience an event that places you or another user in harm's way, please initiate the facility's emergency response system by using the nearest phone and dialing ______________ .

8. In the event of a sudden cardiac event, the Center has an AED located at ______________________________ .

9. No food and drink other than water or sports performance drinks in plastic containers are allowed in this area.

10. Please respect your fellow members by wiping down the equipment when you have finished using it.

11. During peak usage periods, please limit yourself to a maximum of two sets per piece of equipment. If you need to perform more than two sets, please share the equipment with other users in a manner that allows everyone an equal opportunity to pursue their fitness program.

12. Cell phones must be turned off or put on vibrate.

B-3c. Group-Exercise Area Usage Guidelines and Policies

(Name of Center)

Group-Exercise Area Usage Guidelines and Policies

1. Engaging in any form of physical activity carries an increased risk of experiencing an event such as rapid heartbeat, dizziness, orthopedic injury, and in rare instances, stroke, sudden cardiac event, or even death. To minimize these risks, we encourage you to meet with one of the Center's fitness professionals and receive the proper screening and orientation prior to engaging in any exercise.

2. If you have any health condition that would compromise your ability to participate in exercise, please see a fitness professional before participating.

3. We ask that all participants attending group-exercise classes be in the classroom and in position to begin the class at the starting time identified on the group-exercise schedule. Participants who are late to class should warm up prior to entering the class, and when entering the classroom, move to the back of the class so as not to disturb the other participants.

4. The instructor is there to provide instruction, motivation, and most importantly, to provide a safe environment for exercising. We ask that during class, you listen to the instructor and abide by the instructions and counsel given.

5. If, for any reason, you experience difficulty during class, such as dizziness, shortness of breath, experience an injury, feel faint, etc., please cease exercising and let the instructor know of your difficulties. That individual will assist you in receiving the appropriate attention, including, if necessary, initiating the facility's emergency response system by using the nearest phone and dialing ____________________ .

6. In the event of a sudden cardiac event, the Center has an AED located at ____________________________ .

7. The club reserves the right to cancel any classes that average less than ______ participants on a daily basis for a period of 30 days.

8. Cell phones are not allowed in the classroom.

B-3d. Aquatics and Pool Area Usage Guidelines and Policies

(Name of Center)

Aquatics and Pool Area Usage Guidelines and Policies

1. There is no lifeguard on duty. The Center does monitor the pool on a regular basis using ______________, (e.g., surveillance cameras, periodic walk-throughs) but there is no assurance that a staff person will be available to assist you at any given moment. As a result, you are using the pool at your own risk, fully aware that there is no lifeguard on duty at the pool.
2. Please shower before entering the pool.
3. Please do not enter the pool if you have an open wound or other similar condition that might expose bodily fluid to the water.
4. No running or playing around on the pool deck.
5. The pool deck may be slippery due to standing water, so please use caution when walking and moving around on the deck.
6. No diving into the pool.
7. If you experience an emergency and/or witness an emergency, please activate the Center's emergency response system by using the phone located in the pool area and dialing ______________. The following equipment ______, ______, ______, ______ is located in the pool area to assist with an emergency prior to the arrival of those responding to the activation of the emergency response system.
8. Please avoid using any electrical equipment around the pool.
9. No food or drink is allowed in the pool area other than those items indicated below:

   ____

   ____

   ____

   ____

   ____

   ____

   ____

10. Children under the age of 18 who wish to use the pool must be accompanied by a parent or legal guardian at all times.
11. In the event of a sudden cardiac event, the Center has an AED located at ______________________.

B-3e. Locker Room Usage Guidelines and Policies

(Name of Center)
Locker Room Usage Guidelines and Policies

1. Center policy limits children over the age of ______ from entering or using the locker room of the opposite gender. For example, a boy over the age of ______ cannot enter the women's locker room and a girl over the age of ______ cannot enter the men's locker room.
2. Camera phones or any other photography equipment are not allowed in the locker room.
3. The Center is not responsible for personal items left in the locker rooms, including items left in personal lockers.
4. Please be considerate of your fellow members and place all soiled and/or used towels in the designated towel drops.
5. Please be considerate of your fellow members and place all garbage and other used paper products in the designated waste receptacles.
6. Please be aware that the wet areas of the locker room (e.g., showers, rest rooms) present an increased risk of experiencing a slip-and-fall incident due to the presence of water. As a result, caution should be taken when walking in these areas.
7. In the event of a sudden cardiac event, the Center has an AED located at ______________________________ .
8. No food and drink other than water or sports performance drinks in plastic containers are allowed in this area.

Appendix B-4
Sample Professional Staffing Forms

- Employee Development Plan Form
- Employee Performance Objectives—Semi-Annual Form
- New Employee Orientation Checklist
- Compensation Agreement (Salaried Employee)
- Compensation Agreement (Hourly and/or Commission Employee)

The forms in this section are adapted and used with permission from Stephen J. Tharrett and James A. Peterson, *Fitness Management* (2nd Edition). Monterey, CA: Healthy Learning; 2008.

B-4a. Employee Development Plan Form

(Name of Center)

Employee Development Plan Form

This form is designed to provide both management and individual employees with a tool for outlining the annual professional development process for each employee. The objective of incorporating this tool into each employee's overall work experience is to help ensure a structured process of developing each employee's talents for the benefit of the individual employee and the Center.

Employee name: ______________________________

Current position/title: ____________________ Tenure at current position: ____________________

Previous position, if applicable: ____________________ Time in previous position: ____________________

Employee's long-term professional goals:

1. ______________________________
2. ______________________________
3. ______________________________

Employee's professional development goals and action plan for the year: ____________________

Development Goal	Action Step	Target Date

Employee signature: ______________________________

Supervisor signature: ______________________________

Date agreed to: ______________________________

B-4b. Employee Performance Objectives—Semi-Annual Form

(Name of Center)

Employee Performance Objectives—Semi-Annual Form

Employee: ______________________________

Club: ______________________________

Position: ______________________________

Department: ______________________________

Timeframe: ______________________________

The employee and that person's supervisor are to reach agreement on specific performance objectives tied to the employee's job model, which, if achieved, will support the Center's overall business plan objectives. These objectives will then become the framework for conducting the employee's performance evaluation.

#	Performance Objective	Weighting (Percent of Total Job Accountability)	Highest Possible Score
1			
2			
3			
4			
5			

Agreed to by:

Employee signature: ______________________________ Date: ____________

Supervisor signature: ______________________________ Date: ____________

B-4c. New Employee Orientation Checklist

(Name of Center)

New Employee Orientation Checklist

Employee Name: ______________________ Date Hired: ______________________

Employee's Job Title: ______________________ Date Training Begun: ______________________

Center Mentor: ______________________ Center Supervisor: ______________________

Step	Training Activity	Date Completed	Supervisor/ Mentor Initials
1	Go over the employee's job description and compensation agreement with them. Have them sign both. Assign the new employee a mentor.		
2	Review with the employee the Center's Employee Handbook. Have the employee sign the sheet at the end of the handbook when you have finished the review.		
3	Give the new employee a tour of the Center and introduce them to each employee. Make sure to provide the new employee with a list of all employees and their job roles.		
4	Conduct a new user orientation with the employee.		
5	Have the new employee spend time with the sales staff and receive an overview of: • The membership categories and pricing • The Center's process for generating leads • How the Center is different than the competitors Provide the new employee with a new user package.		
6	Have the new employee spend time with the fitness director and receive an overview of : • The Center's personal-training packages and pricing • The Center's philosophy about personal training • Have them observe a trainer working with a member		
7	Have the new employee spend time with the front-desk staff and receive an overview of: • The process for checking in users and guests • The process for scheduling appointments The other general responsibilities of the front-desk receptionist		
8	Have the new employee receive a personal training session.		
9	Have the new employee take a group-exercise class.		
10	Have the new employee spend time with the housecleaning staff and receive an overview of: • The Center's basic cleaning practices • Each employee's role in keeping the Center clean		
11	Complete a 90-day performance plan with the employee and detail specific objectives for them over the first 90 days.		
12	Have the new employee attend the center's new employee orientation class sometime during their first two weeks of work.		
13	Make sure that the new employee is paired with a mentor and receives position-specific training.		
14	Have the new employee complete at least two days of training in the individual's new job, working alongside that person's mentor or another department employee.		

B-4d. Compensation Agreement (Salaried Employee)

(Name of Center)

Compensation Agreement (Salaried Employee)

The undersigned ("You") agree to be employed in the position of ______________________________ by ______________________________ ("the Center"), effective ______________________________, 20______, and to continue such employment for so long as You and the Center both agree. The purpose of this , Agreement is to set forth the Performance Objectives and compensation for this position.

This Agreement is not a contract for employment for a fixed term; instead it describes the terms upon which your compensation is to be based. By signing this Agreement You acknowledge your understanding that either party may terminate the employment relationship at any time, for any reason, with or without cause. The employment-at-will nature of this relationship cannot be altered by any statements, oral or written, made by anyone. Your signature also acknowledges your understanding that compensation does not accrue to You after employment terminates.

1. **Base Fixed Compensation (Salary):** The potential base fixed compensation that can be earned by You on an annualized basis, and the manner and timing of that base fixed compensation, are set forth in Exhibit "A."
2. **Variable Compensation:** The potential variable compensation (e.g. commissions, bonuses) that can be earned by You on an annualized basis, and the manner and timing of that compensation, are set forth in Exhibit "A."
3. **Exempt Position:** Your position as ______________________________ is an exempt position under the minimum wage and overtime provisions of the Fair Labor Standards Act and You are not entitled to overtime compensation. The compensation provided to You shall constitute full payment for services rendered by You to the Center. You shall not receive additional compensation for any services performed unless such services and payment thereof, prior to rendition, are authorized in writing by, or on behalf of, the Center.
4. **Benefits:** Your general benefits are described in the Center's Employee Handbook and any additional benefits for which You may be eligible for are set forth in Exhibit "A."
5. **Duties:** Your duties shall include, but not be limited to, those described in the job description to You and, if applicable, the annual performance goals You receive.
6. **Entire Agreement:** This embodies the entire agreement and understanding of You and the Center relating to your employment and supersedes all prior representations, agreements, and understandings, oral or written, relating to your employment.

Your Name: ______________________________	Center representative: ______________________________
Signature: ______________________________	Signature: ______________________________
Date: ______________________________	Date: ______________________________

B-4d. Compensation Agreement (Salaried Employee) *continued*

Exhibit "A"

1. Base Fixed Compensation:
   a. Compensation period: ______________________________
   b. Compensation amount: ______________________________
   c. Annualized compensation potential: ______________________________

2. Variable Compensation:
   a. Your annual variable compensation potential will be equal to:
   b. Your variable compensation structure (e.g., amount of, method of achievement, and timing of) is as described below:
      ✓ ______________________________
      ✓ ______________________________
      ✓ ______________________________

3. Benefits:
   In addition to the employee benefits described in the Employee Handbook, you are eligible for the following additional benefits:
   a. ______________________________
   b. ______________________________
   c. ______________________________
   d. ______________________________

B-4e. Compensation Agreement (Hourly and/or Commission Employee)

(Name of Center)

Compensation Agreement (Hourly and/or Commission Employee)

The undersigned ("You") agree to be employed in the position of ______________________ by ______________________ ("the Center"), effective ______________, 20____, and shall continue for so long as You and the Center both agree. The purpose of this Agreement is to set forth the Performance Objectives and compensation for this position.

This Agreement is not a contract for employment for a fixed term; instead it describes the terms upon which your compensation is to be based. By signing this Agreement You acknowledge your understanding that either party may terminate the employment relationship at any time, for any reason, with or without cause. The employment-at-will nature of this relationship cannot be altered by any statements, oral or written, made by anyone. You further understand that compensation does not accrue to You after employment terminates.

1. **Hourly Wage:** The hourly wage to be paid to You for fulfilling the accountabilities of your position will be $ ________ per hour for every hour worked to be paid every ______________.
2. **Commission:** You will receive a commission on each class/lesson/session instructed equal to ____ percent (%) of the revenue generated by each class/lesson/session instructed to be paid every __________.
3. **Duties:** Your duties shall include, but not be limited to, those described in your job description and, if applicable, your annual performance goals.
4. **Benefits:** Your general benefits are described in the Center's Employee Handbook.
5. **Entire Agreement:** This embodies the entire agreement and understanding of You and the Center relating to your employment and supersedes all prior representations, agreements, and understandings, oral or written, relating to your employment.

Your Name: ______________________ Center representative: ______________________

Signature: ______________________ Signature: ______________________

Date: ______________________ Date: ______________________

Appendix B-5
Sample Operational Policies and Procedures Forms

- Equipment Maintenance Log Sheet
- Maintenance and Repair Service Request Form
- Opening Report Form

The forms in this section are adapted and used with permission from Stephen J. Tharrett and James A. Peterson, *Fitness Management* (2nd Edition). Monterey, CA: Healthy Learning; 2008.

B-5a. Equipment Maintenance Log Sheet

(Name of Center)

Equipment Maintenance Log Sheet

Basic Information

Name of the piece of equipment:	
Manufacturer of the equipment:	
Serial number:	
Date that installation inspection occurred:	
Date equipment was placed in use:	
Owner's manual check off:	
Location of the owner's manual:	

Service Record

Date of service request	Description of service needed	Staff person taking care of the service	Date service completed	Date equip-ment placed back in use	Staff name and initials

B-5b. Maintenance and Repair Service Request Form

(Name of Center)

Maintenance and Repair Service Request Form

Service order request number: ______________________ Date of request: ______________

Staff person requesting service: ______________________ Position/title: ______________

Signature of staff person requesting service: ______________________

I. Description of Service Being Requested (completed by person requesting service):

1. Area of the facility:	
2. Piece of equipment (if applicable):	
3. Description ofrepair/service/work needed:	
4. When repair/service/work needs to be completed:	Day: ________ Date: ________ Time: ________

Please submit this form to the staff person in charge of facilities and equipment, and keep a record for the files.

II. Results of Request (completed by staff person completing the repair/service/work):

1. Name of staff person completing work:	
2. Day, date, and time work completed:	
3. Signature of staff person completing work:	
4. The quality of the work was:	

After the work is completed, place the form in the appropriate file, and return a copy to the staff person who originally requested the work.

B-5c. Opening Report Form

(Name of Center)
Opening Report

Employee Name: ______________________________ Date: ______________

_______ Turn on lights

_______ Turn on radio; adjust volume; set television on desired channel.

_______ Turn on computer in the fitness testing room and front desk; type in the Center's ID, date, and day of the week

_______ Set up control desk:

- _______ Pull out appointment book and turn to correct date
- _______ Check on message from previous night
- _______ Sharpen pencils if needed
- _______ Rip day off of small calendar

_______ Check out locker rooms and make sure they are clean, and supplies are replenished; roll out shower mats

_______ Check out the fitness floor and make sure all equipment is turned on and ready to go

_______ Put away uniform bags

_______ Fold towels

_______ Put load in dryer

_______ Read MOD log

_______ Unlock concessions case

_______ Check tires on Velodyne

_______ Check all offices, aerobic room, and both locker rooms

_______ Check strength fitness area for footprints and note in MOD book

_______ Call and check on the specific time before opening

_______ Check all clocks before opening

_______ Check temperature throughout club (thermostats on 68 degrees)

_______ Make sure no light bulbs are burned out

_______ Check ceiling tiles for leaks

_______ Walk entire perimeter of the Center

_______ Check schedule and note activities, special events, and massage appointments

_______ Turn on copier

_______ Write cleaning inspection notes in log book

Appendix B-6
Sample Quality Management Forms

- Strategic Planning Worksheet
- Strategic Plan Action Worksheet
- Program Best Practices Benchmark Form
- User Feedback Form
- Tracking Operating Performance Form

The forms in this section are adapted and used with permission from Stephen J. Tharrett and James A. Peterson, *Fitness Management* (2nd Edition). Monterey, CA: Healthy Learning; 2008.

B-6a. Strategic Planning Worksheet

(Name of Center)
Strategic Planning Worksheet

I. Mission (whom do you serve, what is the Center's product, how do you deliver it and its value)

II. Vision (what is it that you want the Center to be in 3-5 years)

III. Promise (what is it that you want the user and/or employee to always experience)

B-6a. Strategic Planning Worksheet *continued*

IV. Core Values (the roots for every decision and action you take)

1	
2	
3	
4	
5	

V. Objectives & Goals (what is it you want the Center to achieve and target)

Audience/Target	Objectives

B-6a. Strategic Planning Worksheet *continued*

(Name of Center)
Strategic Planning Worksheet

VI. Strategies (the guidelines and general actions that will lead to achievement of the objectives)

Objective	Specific Strategies	Outcome Measures	Person Responsible

B-6b. Strategic Plan Action Worksheet

(Name of Center)
Strategic Plan Action Worksheet

Objective:			
Target #:		**Timline:**	
Strategy:			

#	Action Steps	Leader

B-6c. Program Best Practices Benchmark Form

(Name of Center)
Program Best Practices Benchmark Form

Center Name: ____________________ Contact Name: ____________________

Telephone: ____________________ Fax: ____________________

Email: ____________________

I. Program Title:

II. Program Overview (limit one paragraph):

III Program Specifics:

A. Program Goals

B. Equipment/Facility Needs

C. Number of Members/Guests Participating (if personal training list # sessions weekly and % of total membership)

B-6c. Program Best Practices Benchmark Form *continued*

D. Marketing/Promotion Actions (list specific actions you took to market the program and sign-up of participants

1	
2	
3	
4	
5	

E. Number of Staff Involved

IV. Participant Feedback and Opportunities for Improvement:

V. Revenue & Expense = Profitability:

Revenues		Expenses & Net	
# Participants		Payroll	
Fee Charged		Commissions	
Revenue from Fees		Other Expenses	
Other Revenue (sponsor)		Total Expenses	
Total Revenue		Program Net	

VI. The Five Keys That MADE IT WORK:

1	
2	
3	
4	
5	

Please attach any marketing materials or related materials used in delivering and marketing your program.

B-6d. User Feedback Form

(Name of Center)
Share Your Experience

Member & Guest Comment Card

Date: ______________________ Time: ______________________

Experiences you would like to share:

Overall, how did you feel about your experience in the Center today? Please indicate by checking the appropriate response:

- ❑ Unsatisfactory (did not meet my expectations)
- ❑ Satisfactory (met my expectations and needs)
- ❑ Delighted (exceeded my expectations, wow)

Would you like us to follow up with you directly? ❑ Yes ❑ No

If yes, please provide your name and contact information.

Name (optional): ____

Contact phone #: ______________________ Contact e-mail: ______________________

______________________ ______________________

Thank you for sharing your feelings about your experience today.

B-6e. Tracking Operating Performance Form

(Name of Center)
Tracking Operating Performance

Using industry benchmarks to compare a medical fitness center's performance against others in the industry can be an important way to measure and identify potential opportunities to improve operational performance. However, it is important to note that benchmark data represent averages for centers, not just the best performing facilities. The goals, objectives, and performance of centers may vary significantly due to the need to focus on different populations and member mix (employees, seniors, families, and those with special health needs), varying levels of comprehensiveness (types of facility amenities and variety of programming), size, and affluence of the market, among other factors.

While benchmarking can be helpful, it is more important for an organization to track its own experience over time, and with specific goals and objectives in mind than to track its performance against the average facility. The following list details several important variables to track internally, as well as measure against industry benchmarks. Ideally, all data should be captured and monitored on a monthly basis to identify trends before they become problematic and to recognize opportunities and challenges that need to be addressed.

Scorecard: Tracking Operating Performance

A. ❑ *USER DATA*

Forecast	Actual	
______	______	• Total number of members (individuals)
______	______	• Total membership accounts by type of membership (e.g., individual, couple, family, employee, senior, corporate)
______	______	• Square feet/member
______	______	• Number of prospective members who visited the facility
______	______	• New members enrolled
______	______	• Sales conversion % (percent of prospects who become members)
______	______	• Member terminations
______	______	• Member attrition % (terminations as percent of beginning number of members)
______	______	• Net membership growth rate
______	______	• Medical referrals in (members referred *from* clinical services or physicians)
______	______	• Medical referrals out (members referred *to* clinical services or physicians)
______	______	• Total member visits/week
______	______	• Total member visits/week/sq ft
______	______	• Percentage of active members to total members (active defined as using the center an average of 4 times per month)
______	______	• Total number of participants by type of program (e.g., exercise classes, personal training, wellness education, camps, etc.)

B-6e. Tracking Operating Performance Form *continued*

B. ❑ *REVENUE/EXPENSE DATA*

Budgeted Actual

______ ______ • Total revenues
______ ______ • Dues revenue % of total revenues
______ ______ • Non-dues revenue % of total revenues
______ ______ • Revenue/square foot
______ ______ • Revenue/member
______ ______ • Revenue/FTE
______ ______ • Total expenses
______ ______ • Payroll & benefits
______ ______ • Personnel costs % of total revenues
______ ______ • Number of FTEs
______ ______ • Number of employees (full-time, part-time, contract if assigned hours)
______ ______ • Members/FTE
______ ______ • Marketing costs
______ ______ • Marketing cost per new member
______ ______ • Net operating margin (total revenues less total expenses)
______ ______ • Operating margin % of total revenues
______ ______ • Bad debts % of total revenues

Appendix C
Trade and Professional Associations Involved in Medical Fitness, Health, and Related Wellness Concerns

Aerobics and Fitness Association of America
15250 Ventura Boulevard, Suite 200
Sherman Oaks, CA 91403
877-968-7263
www.afaa.com

American Academy of Physical Medicine and Rehabilitation
One IBM Plaza, Suite 2500
Chicago, IL 60611-3604
312-464-9700
www.aapmr.org

American Association of Cardiovascular and Pulmonary Rehabilitation
401 North Michigan Avenue, Suite 2200
Chicago, IL 60611
312-321-5146
www.aacvpr.org

American Alliance for Health, Physical Education, Recreation and Dance
1900 Association Drive
Reston, VA 20191
800-213-7193
www.aahperd.org

American College of Sports Medicine
401 West Michigan Street
P.O. Box 1440
Indianapolis, IN 42606-1440
317-637-9200
www.acsm.org

American Council on Exercise
4851 Paramount Drive
San Diego, CA 92123
800-825-3636
www.acefitness.org

American Heart Association
7272 Greenville Avenue
Dallas, TX 75231
800-242-8721
www.americanheart.org

American Massage Therapy Association
500 Davis Street, Suite 900
Evanston, IL 60201-4444
877-905-2700
www.amta-wa.org

American Society for Testing and Materials International
100 Barr Harbor Drive
P.O. Box C700
West Conshohocken, PA 19428-2959
www.astm.org

Barrier Free Environments, Inc.
P.O. Box 30634
Highway 70 West-Watergarden
Raleigh, NC 27622
919-782-7823

Cooper Institute
12330 Preston Road
Dallas, TX 75230
1-972-341-3200
www.cooperinst.org

Centers for Medicare and Medicaid Services
7500 Security Boulevard
Baltimore, MD, 21244
www.cms.hhs.gov
For cardiac rehab coverage:
http://www.cms.hhs.gov/Transmittals/Downloads/R52NCD.pdf

IDEA Health & Fitness Association
10455 Pacific Center Ct.
San Diego, CA. 92121-4339
800-999-4332
www.ideafit.com

International Fitness Professionals Association
14509 University Point Place
Tampa, FL 33613
1-800-785-1924
www.ifpa-fitness.com

International Health, Racquet and Sportsclub Association
70 Fargo Street
Boston, MA 02210
800-228-4772
www.ihrsa.org

National Academy of Sports Medicine
26632 Agoura Road
Calabasas, CA 91302
www.nasm.org

National Athletic Trainers Association
2952 Stemmons Freeway
Dallas, TX 75247
214-637-6282
www.nata.org

National Center on Physical Activity and Disability
1640 W. Roosevelt Road
Chicago, IL 60608-6904
1-800-900-8086
www.ncpad.org

National Commission for Certifying Agencies
2025 M Street, N.W., Suite 800
Washington, DC 20036
1-202-367-1165
www.noca.org

National Diabetes Education Program
One Diabetes Way
Bethesda, MD 20814-9692
1-301-496-3583
www.ndep.nih.gov

National Institute for Occupational Safety and Health
Hubert Humphrey Building
200 Independence Avenue, SW
Washington, DC 20201
800-356-4674
www.cdc.gov/niosh

National Strength and Conditioning Association
1885 Bob Johnson Drive
Colorado Springs, CO 80906
800-815-6826
www.nsca-lift.org

National Swimming Pool Association
4775 Granby Circle
Colorado Springs, CO 80919-3131
719-540-9119
www.nspf.com

National Wellness Institute
1300 College Court
P.O. Box 827
Stevens Point, WI 54481
800-243-8694
www.nationalwellness.org

President's Council on Physical Fitness and Sports
200 Independence Avenue, SW, Room 738-H
Washington, DC 20201-0004
202-690-9000
www.fitness.gov

Wellness Councils of America
9802 Nicholas Street, Suite 315
Omaha, NE 68114
402-827-3590
www.welcoa.org

Appendix D
Suggested References

American Association for Cardiovascular and Pulmonary Rehabilitation. *AACVPR Guidelines for Cardiac Rehabilitation and Secondary Prevention Programs. 4th Edition.* Champaign, IL: Human Kinetics; 2004.

American College of Sports Medicine. *ACSM's Guidelines for Exercise Testing and Prescription. 7th Edition.* Philadelphia: Lippincott, Williams and Wilkins; 2006.

American College of Sports Medicine. *ACSM's Health and Fitness Facility Standards and Guidelines. 3rd Edition.* Champaign, IL: Human Kinetics; 2007.

American College of Sports Medicine and American Heart Association. *Joint position statement on automated external defibrillators in health/fitness facilities.* 2002.

American Heart Association and American College of Sports Medicine. Joint statement: Recommendations for cardiovascular screening, staffing and emergency policies at health/fitness facilities. *Circulation* 30(6): 1-19. 1998.

American Heart Association. Guidelines 2000 for cardiopulmonary resuscitation and emergency cardiovascular care. *Supplement to Circulation* 102(8): August 2000.

Barry, Robert, Amy C. Murcko, and Clifford E. Brubaker. *The Six Sigma Book for Healthcare: Improving Outcomes by Reducing Errors.* Chicago, IL: Health Administration Press; 2002.

Canadian Society for Exercise Physiology. Recommendations for the fitness assessment, programming, and counseling of persons with a disability. *Canadian Journal of Applied Physiology.* (23)3: 119-130. 1998.

Collins, James C. and Jerry Porras. *Build to Last: Successful Habits of Visionary Companies.* New York: Harper-Collins Publishers, Inc.; 1994.

England, Hannah, Hanna Weinberg, et al. The automated external defibrillator: Clinical benefits and legal liability. *JAMA.* (295)6: 687-690. February 8, 2006.

Haskell, William L., I-Min Lee, Russell R. Pate, et al. Physical Activity and Public Health: Updated Recommendation for Adults from the American College of Sports Medicine and the American Heart Association. MSSE. Vol. 39, No. 8, 1423-1434, 2007.

Herbert, David L.; Herbert, W.G. *Legal Aspects of Preventive, Rehabilitative and Recreational Exercise Programs. 4th Edition.* Canton, OH: PRC Publishing; 2002.

International Health, Racquet and Sportclub Association. *Health and Safety, Legal and Ethical Standards for U.S. IHRSA Clubs: Standards Facilitation Guide.* Boston: 1998.

King, Marjorie L., et al. Medical director responsibilities for outpatient cardiac rehabilitation/secondary prevention programs: A statement for healthcare professionals from the American Association for Cardiovascular and Pulmonary Rehabilitation and the American Heart Association. *Journal of Cardiopulmonary Rehabilitation.* (25)6: 315-319. Nov/Dec 2005.

Nelson, Miriam E., W. Jack Rejeski, Steven N. Blair, et al. Physical activity and public health in older adults: Recommendation from the American College of Sports Medicine and the American Heart Association. *MSSE.* (39) 8: 1435-1445. 2007.

Ransom, Scott B., Maulik S. Joshi and David B. Nash (editors). *The Healthcare Quality Book: Vision, Strategy, and Tools.* Chicago, IL: Health Administration Press; 2005.

United States Access Board. *Accessible sports facilities: A summary of accessibility guidelines for recreation facilities.* Supplement to Americans with Disabilities Act Access Guidelines. 2002.

United States Access Board. *Accessible swimming pools and spas: A summary of accessibility guidelines for recreation facilities.* Supplement to Americans with Disabilities Act Access Guidelines. 2002.

United States Department of Health and Human Services. 2008 Physical Activity Guidelines for Americans. www.health.gov/paguidelines ODPHP Publication No. U0036, Oct 2008.

Tharrett, Stephen J. *The ACE Fitness and Business Forms Handbook.* Monterey, CA: Healthy Learning; 2006

Tharrett, Stephen J. *The Health Fitness Club Operator's Guide to Recruiting and Retaining Great Employees.* Monterey, CA: Healthy Learning; 2007

Tharrett, Stephen J. and James A. Peterson. *Fitness Management. 2nd Edition.* Monterey, CA: Healthy Learning; 2008

Appendix E
Meeting The Roadmap for Excellence: A Standards/Guidelines Checklist for Medical Fitness Center Facilities

I. Medical Oversight

Standard 1: A Medical Fitness Center must have medical oversight.

Guideline		Yes	No
1.1	Does the facility have a medical director, physician advisory committee, or physician advisor in place?		
1.1a	Does the facility medical leadership and the medical director/advisory committee meet at least four times per year?		
1.1b	Does the medical director and/or advisory committee provide oversight of the facility for:		
	a. emergency response/code policy/procedure review?		
	b. facility's AED program?		
	c. staff emergency response training?		
	d. periodic review of emergency/code response, outcomes and identification of opportunities for improvement?		
	e. periodic review of clinical policies?		
	f. periodic review of initial and ongoing screening programs?		
	g. program content and special populations?		
1.2	Does the medical leadership encourage cross-training efforts for rehabilitation programs?		
1.3	Does the medical leadership assist in the development of clinical program content and safety considerations for special populations?		

Standard 2: The clinical programs/services offered within a Medical Fitness Center must comply with the current requirements of the Centers for Medicare and Medicare Services.

Guideline		Yes	No
2.1	Are the requirements of the Centers for Medicare and Medicaid Services reviewed periodically?		
2.2	Are the results of the review recorded and evaluated to determine whether subsequent action should be undertaken?		

Standard 3: A Medical Fitness Center must demonstrate a direct and valid relationship with its community healthcare system/local continuum of healthcare.

Guideline		Yes	No
3.1	Does the facility's mission statement include a commitment by the facility to participate in the local continuum of healthcare?		
3.2	Does the facility maintain, for at least one year, documentation of its involvement in the local continuum of healthcare?		
3.3	Does the facility maintain records of its involvement in:		
	a. maintaining ownership by a hospital, health system and/or a physician/physician group?		
	b. referral patterns to and from phsyicians and/or physician extenders for clinical services provided by the facility?		
	c. hosted community and professional education programs/seminars on health-related topics?		
	d. health-related screenings and associated results and follow-up for individuals who have results outside of the normal or expected range?		

II. Pre-Activity Screening

Standard 4: A Medical Fitness Center must offer each member an appropriate pre-activity screening process, and refer moderate- to high-risk individuals to their respective physician for medical clearance prior to participation.

Guideline		Yes	No
4.1	Does the facility have a systematic process of screening for chronic diseases, associated risk stratification, and the participant's potential for exercise-related injury?		
4.2	Are all pre-activity screening procedures straightforward, easy-to-understand, and conducted in a time-efficient manner? Is every feasible step undertaken to encourage all users to engage in the pre-screening process?		
4.3	Are all facility users offered a pre-activity screening prior to their participation in physical activities at the facility? If a user should decline the pre-activity screening, is that person permitted to sign a waiver for the screening that allows that individual to participate in the program offerings of the facility?		

Guideline

		Yes	No
4.4	Does the waiver for an individual who refuses to participate in the pre-activity screening clearly delineate that the person has been offered a pre-activity screening, has been informed of the basic risks involved in participating, has chosen not to follow the guidance provided by the facility's staff, has assumed responsibility for his/her own actions, and has released the facility from any legal responsibility from claims or suits arising from his/her participation in the facility's programs?		

Standard 5: If the pre-activity screening identifies a potential user as having a known cardiovascular, metabolic, or pulmonary disease and/or is identified as a high-risk individual, the user should be advised, in writing, to consult with a physician and/or qualified healthcare provider, and provide documentation of such consult to the facility prior to participating in physical activity at the facility.

Guideline

		Yes	No
5.1	Are all facility users who are identified as having risk factors that necessitate referral for medical consultation, who fail to obtain such consultation, permitted to sign a waiver that allows them to participate in the program offerings of the facility?		
5.2	To the extent permitted by law, are such users who refuse to sign the waiver precluded from participating in the program activities of the facility?		

Standard 6: The pre-activity screen should be reviewed and interpreted by qualified staff and the results documented, including referral to a qualified healthcare provider and the outcome of such consultation.

Guideline

		Yes	No
6.1	Are the results of the pre-activity screening utilized to identify and make appropriate decisions about what constitutes safe activity levels and modalities for that particular person?		
6.2	Consistent with the Health Insurance Portability and Accountability Act of 1996 (HIPAA), is a form that details a user's health information and offers a means for explicitly recording medical clearance (if given by appropriate medical professional) provided by the facility to the individual to take to a physician?		

III. Risk Management & Emergency-Response Policies

Standard 7: The Medical Fitness Center must have a written emergency-response plan that enables a timely and appropriate response to any emergency that threatens the health and safety of facility users.

Guideline		Yes	No
7.1	Does the emergency-response plan specify the most likely emergency situations that could occur and how each circumstance will be handled, including the precise responsibilities of the first, second, and third responders to a particular emergency?		
7.2	Is the emergency-response plan fully detailed in writing and maintained in an area easily accessed by facility staff? Does the plan also include procedures for documenting in writing the fact that the emergency-response system is reviewed on a regular basis by every member of the facility's staff?		
7.3	Does the facility have a prompt and direct link to the "911" emergency-response center? Are staff members made aware of the locations for all emergency equipment, including the facility's telephones?		
7.4	Does the facility have an adequate number of first-aid kits and other necessary emergency equipment, including documentation that all equipment is periodically checked for functionality?		
7.5	Does the facility hold regular emergency drills (e.g., at least four times a year) and maintain associated documentation that demonstrates the competencies of staff to respond to emergency situations?		
7.6	Does the facility have a formal incident reporting and management program in place?		
7.7	Does the facility have signs and information in place to alert facility users to the emergency-response system?		
7.8	Was the emergency-response plan developed in concert with the local emergency medical services (EMS) provider in the area of the facility?		

Standard 8: With physician oversight in place, a Medical Fitness Center must have an appropriate number of automatic external defibrillators (AEDs) that are easily accessible for use.

Guideline		Yes	No
8.1	Is the number of AEDs and the placement of the AEDs in a facility appropriate for the response time/distance (within 1.5 minute walk) to any potential location in the facility that it could be needed?		
8.2	Does all staff have current CPR/AED training?		
8.3	Is each AED maintained according to the manufacturer's guidelines and is maintenance and monitoring documentation kept current?		
8.4	Are review and practice sessions conducted on a periodic basis (e.g., once every three months) to ensure that all facility staff possess the appropriate skills for safely using an AED?		

Standard 9: A Medical Fitness Center with aquatics areas must have specific written emergency plans for each pool.

Guideline		Yes	No
9.1	Have written policies and procedures been developed that specify the responsibilities of staff for handling emergencies in the aquatics areas of the facility, including the role of first, second, and third responder?		
9.2	Are staff provided with regular training opportunities for water-related emergencies, with associated documentation that demonstrates the competencies of staff to respond in an appropriate manner to aquatics-emergency situations?		
9.3	Is a review of the emergency system for responding to emergencies in the aquatics areas of the facility periodically undertaken to ensure that the policies and procedures are appropriate and are fully understood by staff?		
9.4	Do all aquatics staff and volunteers conducting programs and activities in the facility 's aquatics areas meet the criteria established by the YMCA for such personnel?		
9.5	Has the facility taken documented steps to warn users of actions that pose potential risks to their health and safety, including head-first entry, breath-holding, and underwater swimming?		
9.6	Has the facility developed and implemented specific policies that guarantee adequate supervision of children who seven years old or less while they're in aquatics areas?		
9.7	Has the facility developed a policy and procedures for handling fecal-accidents in aquatics areas?		
9.8	Has the facility developed a detailed plan to minimize the risk of potential entrapments and entanglements in the aquatics areas?		

IV. Programs and Services

Standard 10: A Medical Fitness Center must have programs and services that address the needs and interests of its users.

Guideline		Yes	No
10.1	Does the facility have programs for persons with chronic medical conditions, such as heart disease (CAD, CHF), pulmonary disease, cancer, chronic pain, orthopedic and/or neurologic problems (e.g., arthritis, fibromyalgia, osteoporosis, MS), cerebrovascular disease (stroke), sports injury prevention and rehabilitation, nutritional counseling, etc.?		
10.2	Are all treatments/interventions for facility participants based on and adhere to nationally accepted guidelines?		
10.3	Does each program have appropriate inclusion and exclusion criteria?		
10.4	Do participants undergo a documented initial assessment, with a follow-up reporting to the referring physician and/or healthcare provider?		
10.5	Do programs provide nutritional counseling by qualified staff, when appropriate?		

Guideline		Yes	No
10.6	Is appropriate mental-health counseling available to clinical program participants, as necessary, either provided by the facility, through the participant's primary-care physician, and/or by referral to a mental-health provider?		
10.7	Does the facility offer educational workshops/classes for clinical program participants, and, when appropriate, family members?		
10.8	Do staff maintain an open line of communication when referring physicians and other medical providers to provide members with optimal care and programming? Is a periodic follow-up with referring healthcare providers and/or primary-care providers, as appropriate, encouraged and documented?		
10.9	Does the facility have policies and procedures in place that protect the confidentiality of all patients/clients and comply with all HIPAA standards of privacy and confidentiality for medical information?		
10.10	Does the facility have educational workshops/classes in place for the community that utilize healthcare professionals from the community, as well as staff expertise?		
10.11	Does the facility have lifestyle modification programs that are available for members and the community at large?		

Standard 11: A Medical Fitness Center with aquatics facilities must have written policies and procedures specific to the programs and services that are to be offered in each aquatics area.

Guideline		Yes	No
11.1	Does the facility have aquatics policies and procedures in place that include, but are not limited to, basic rules/regulations for pool use, emergency procedures, and pool and program/class supervision guidelines?		

V. Professional Staffing

Standard 12: Qualifications. A Medical Fitness Center must employ one or more professional(s) who hold degree(s), certification(s), and/or license(s) appropriate to each program offered and the population served

Guideline		Yes	No
12.1	Do fitness directors, managers, or supervisors hold the following minimum qualifications?		
	a. education: bachelor's degree in exercise science or related field; master's degree preferred?		
	b. certification: current fitness instructor, personal trainer, or higher certification that is accredited by the NCCA?		
12.2	Do fitness instructors/staff hold the following minimum qualifications?		
	a. education: college certificate or associate's degree in exercise science; bachelor's degree in exercise science or related field preferred?		
	b. certification: fitness instructor, personal trainer certification, or its equivalent that is accredited by the NCCA?		

Guideline		Yes	No
12.3	Do personal training staff hold the following minimum qualifications?		
	a. education: college certificate or associate's degree; bachelor's degree in exercise science or related field preferred?		
	b. certification: fitness instructor, personal trainer certification, or its equivalent that is accredited by the NCAA?		
12.4	Do clinical fitness staff providing programming for special populations hold the following additional qualifications: ❑ Cardiopulmonary rehabilitation and/or other chronic disease program:		
	a. education: bachelor's degree in exercise science or related field; master's degree preferred?		
	b. certification/licensure: professional NCCA-accredited clinical certification and/or licensed RN or PT with exercise science background; or, for pulmonary rehabilitation, licensed RT?		
	c. experience/training: additional training and/or credential specific to the target population?		
	❑ Orthopedic rehabilitation/post-rehabilitation:		
	a. education: bachelor's degree in exercise science, physical therapy, or athletic training; master's degree preferred?		
	b. certification/licensure: professional clinical certification that is NCCA accredited and/or licensed RN, PT assistant, PT, or ATC?		
	❑ Weight loss:		
	a. education: bachelor's degree in nutrition; additional course work or degree in exercise science preferred?		
	b. certification/licensure: RD license preferred; NCCA-accredited certification (e.g., fitness instructor or personal trainer) and specialty certificate in nutrition/weight loss?		
	c. staff maintain compliance with specific state practice act?		
12.5	Do group-exercise instructors hold the following minimum qualifications:		
	a. education: college certificate or associate's degree in fitness/exercise science; bachelor's degree in exercise science or related field preferred?		
	b. certification: group-exercise instructor or leader certification that is NCCA accredited?		
	c. certificate of completion or specialty certificates from a reputable organization for each specialized group modality that the instructor teaches (e.g., spinning/group cycling)?		
12.6	Does the aquatics director/supervisor hold the following minimum qualifications:		
	a. education: college certificate or associate's degree in fitness/exercise science; bachelor's degree in exercise science, recreation, or related field preferred?		
	b. certification: current YMCA and/or Red Cross certification; certification as an aquatics facility operator; certification as a pool operator, advanced life-saving certification, and/or water safety instructor certification?		
12.7	Do aquatics staff hold the following minimum qualifications:		
	a. certification: appropriate aquatics certification or specialty training certificate for position/responsibilities (e.g., lifeguard, swim instructor, WSI, aquatics exercise instructor)?		

Standard 13: All staff must maintain a current certificate in automated external defibrillation (AED) and cardiopulmonary resuscitation (CPR) from a qualified certifying organization.

Guideline		Yes	No
13.1	Does the facility provide a specific opportunity (i.e., expenses reimbursed, release time, etc.) for each staff member to obtain an AED/CPR certificate?		
13.2	Does the facility have a procedure to ensure that every staff member's AED/CPR certificate is current?		
13.3	Does the facility provide professional liability insurance liability insurance for staff and/or encourage staff to maintain individual policies?		

Standard 14: Staff Training/Continuing Education. A Medical Fitness Center must provide a variety of training/continuing education opportunities for staff, utilizing relationships with and the expertise of, physicians, other community healthcare professionals and/or experts, conferences, and distance-learning programs that are approved for CECs.

Guideline		Yes	No
14.1	Does the facility provide one or more of the following for each professional staff member:		
	a. periodic travel/educational opportunities for staff to attend conferences, observe seminars, make site visits, etc.?		
	b. facility-sponsored workshops, seminars, and conferences for staff and other health professionals?		
	c. current literature resources/medical library access?		
	d. web-based/online training opportunities?		

Standard 15: A Medical Fitness Center must demonstrate that all staff maintain current certification(s)/license(s) by meeting the continuing education requirements for their specific certifying/licensing bodies.

Guideline		Yes	No
15.1	Do all certified and/or licensed professional fitness staff maintain the following:		
	a. current NCCA-accredited certification/license?		
	b. current CPR/AED card?		
	c. annual Universal Precautions training?		
15.3	Does the facility have a process in place to ensure that all staff credentials are current?		

VI. Operational Policies and Practices

Standard 16: A Medical Fitness Center must have a system in place that accurately monitors who has entered and remains in the facility at any given time.

Guideline		Yes	No
16.1	Has the facility implemented a procedure to ensure that every individual in the facility has appropriate access privileges?		
16.2	Are all guests and visitors required to check-in?		
16.3	Are all non-authorized users required to either complete a pre-activity screening instrument or sign a waiver?		
16.4	Is the number of staff scheduled to be present in the facility adjusted, as appropriate, in response to the usage-rate data?		

Standard 17: A Medical Fitness Center must have a system in place for helping ensure that every user achieves the maximum benefits of their exercise and program participant efforts.

Guideline		Yes	No
17.1	Does the facility employ accepted methods to assess functional capacity, body composition, muscular fitness, flexibility, balance, and other components of physical and motor fitness:		
	a. Does the facility offer exercise testing for fitness assessments, as well as for exercise prescription purposes?		
	b. Is all fitness testing conducted and interpreted by qualified staff, according to industry accepted methods/protocols?		
17.2	Does the facility utilize the results of a user's fitness testing as a starting point for developing an appropriate exercise prescription for that individual and as a basis for monitoring progress in the program?		
17.3	Are all facility users offered an initial orientation to the facility, facility equipment, basic program concepts, and emergency/safety guidelines?		

Standard 18: A Medical Fitness Center must comply with all local, state, and federal laws and regulations governing the operation of their facility including—but not limited to—building codes, ADA, OHSA, etc.

Guideline		Yes	No
18.1	Does the facility have an appropriate level of air circulation and air quality?		
18.2	Does the facility have an appropriate level of illumination to help ensure that a reasonably safe environment for engaging in physical activity exists?		
18.3	Does the facility have a reasonable amount of access space between equipment and activity areas?		
18.4	Does the facility separate activity areas from spaces devoted to maintenance, storage, and front-of-the-house and back-of-the-house operations?		

Guideline		Yes	No
18.5	Does the facility have an appropriate number of restrooms?		
18.6	Does the facility have wall and floor surfaces in its activity areas that minimize the risk of injury to participants?		
18.7	Is the facility accessible to disabled individuals?		
18.8	Is facility equipment inclusive to allow the majority of the disabled access to a full-body workout?		
18.9	Does the facility provide staff with training that augments their understanding of the needs of the disabled and various age groups, such as children and the elderly?		
18.10	Does the facility annually conduct an accessibility survey utilizing disabled persons and document efforts to enhance facility accessibility?		
18.11	Does the facility conduct preventative maintenance on all of its exercise equipment according to guidelines provided by the equipment's manufacturer? Is a written record of the maintenance inspection and follow-up kept for at least a year? Are all safety concerns involving equipment in the facility appropriately addressed in a timely manner?		

Standard 19: A Medical Fitness Center with aquatics facilities must comply with all local and state laws/regulations regarding pool chemistry, chemical storage, pool supervision, signage, etc.

Guideline		Yes	No
19.1	Does the facility employ or contract with at least one staff person who is a certified pool operator (CPO)?		
19.2	Is the pool chemistry checked on a regular basis, as required by state/local regulations, and is the documentation recorded?		
19.3	Is signage posted in easily viewed areas and include pool user rules/regulations, appropriate warnings, and emergency procedures?		
19.4	Does the facility maintain and follow a written fecal-accident policy and educate users regarding the importance of following pool hygiene rules?		
19.5	Are pool chemicals stored in appropriately secured locations and in a manner consistent with state laws and regulations?		
19.6	Are material safety data sheet(s) (MSDS) posted and/or available in the aquatics chemical storage area, and be readily obtainable by all staff members?		

Standard 20: A Medical Fitness Center must meet all current local code, state, and OSHA requirements for potentially hazardous materials, including handling of bodily fluids.

Guideline		Yes	No
20.1	Are material safety data sheets, for each potentially hazardous material, maintained and readily available to all staff members? Do staff members receive regular training/review in the handling of potentially hazardous materials, at least on an annual basis?		
20.2	Does the facility provide and document staff training regarding the appropriate handling of bodily fluids and cleaning of contaminated surfaces?		
20.3	Does the facility conduct and document a safety audit at regular intervals and review the results with the medical director or medical advisory committee?		

VII. Signage

Standard 21: A Medical Fitness Center must conspicuously post the appropriate signage indicating caution, danger, and warning in those locations that warrant such signage.

Guideline		Yes	No
21.1	Does the facility post signage that alerts users that a specific activity may expose them to an increased levels of risk in every activity area (e.g., sauna, steam room, whirlpool, aquatics, racquet courts, fitness area, etc.) in which such signage is appropriate?		
21.2	Does the facility post signage in the fitness area that informs users about the need for and how to utilize perceived exertion charts or target heart rate charts for monitoring levels of exertion while exercising?		
21.3	Does the facility post signage about hazardous conditions in the facility or when equipment is out of order?		
21.4	Does such signage have the required signal icon, signal word, signal color, and layout, as specified by the American National Standards Institute (ANSI)?		

Standard 22: A Medical Fitness Center must post all required ADA and OSHA signage.

Guideline		Yes	No
22.1	Does the facility provide signage that indicates access points for individuals with physical challenges?		
22.2	Does the facility provide signage that can be viewed by those individuals who have impaired vision?		
22.3	Does the facility provide signage that informs individuals of the possible exposure to hazardous chemicals and blood-borne chemicals?		

Standard 23: A Medical Fitness Center must post signage involving fire and related emergency situations, as required by local, state, and federal regulations and codes.

Guideline		Yes	No
23.1	Does the facility post signage indicating certificate of occupancy?		
23.2	Does the facility post emergency exit signage?		
23.3	Does the facility post signage indicating the location of emergency phone(s), fire extinguisher(s), AED units, and first-aid equipment?		
23.4	Does the facility work closely with its local fire department and city officials to ensure that it is in complete compliance with the requirement for fire and emergency situation signage?		

VIII. Quality Management

Standard 24: A Medical Fitness Center must have a systematic process in place to continuously assess and improve all aspects of health and fitness delivery, including, but not limited to, individual user outcomes, clinical and non-clinical programs/services, and operational/business processes.

Guideline		Yes	No
24.1	Does the facility have a policy and procedure in place for ensuring that all activities involving a particular program/service/process are effective and efficient, with respect to expectations and the facility's mission, stated goals, and objectives?		
24.2	Does the facility's quality management program provide coordination, integration, and support for performance-improvement activities throughout the center and ensure participation by all departments and services in order to help accomplish the following:		
	a. achieve a collaborative process in the design of new services, programs, or processes?		
	b. identify and utilize key findings to improve performance, key processes, and member/patient/user experience and safety?		
	c. minimize delays, errors, and rework in providing services by focusing improvement efforts on the well-planned, cost-effective, and service-oriented progression of each individual through the health and fitness experience?		
	d. assure communication and reporting among facility administration, physicians and other healthcare providers, managers/supervisors, staff, and medical directory/advisory committees?		
	e. provide for rapid identification and prevention of adverse user experiences, and facilitate optimal management through coordination of appropriate responses?		
	f. identify and address user/patient, partner, and community needs in accordance with the facility's mission?		

Guideline		Yes	No
24.3	Does the facility's quality-management program provide for regular reporting, oversight, and publishing of performance improvement activities and associated results, such as:		
	a. general program and individual member results and outcomes?		
	b. compliance with stated goals, including major reasons for successes and failures?		
	c. reason(s) for the termination of program(s)?		
	e. key implemented projects designed to improve performance?		
24.4	Does the facility have a standardized method of measuring and evaluating the output/outcome of programs, procedures, and processes and for modifying each, based on the results, to increase its effectiveness and performance? Are facility goals and objectives and state, regional, and/or national data, if available, used as benchmarks during the process?		
24.5	Are performance improvement/outcome data measured, evaluated, acted upon, and documented, including:		
	a. safety/emergency-response/sentinel events		
	b. individual member/user outcomes, such as referrals to and from physicians and healthcare providers, pre-activity screenings, expanded health-risk appraisals, fitness testing/evaluations, and exercise and other risk factors/lifestyle-change programming		
	c. facility programs, such as clinical and non-clinical programs/services, health-		
	related seminars/classes/programs, and health-related screenings		
	d. surveys, such as member satisfaction, patient satisfaction, seminar/class/program, and employee satisfaction		
	e. business processes and performance		
	f. benchmarks/standards of the facility's operational performance, including operating margin, labor as a percentage of revenue, volumes (e.g., visits, programs, etc.), FTEs, FTE and/or salary per unit (e.g., visit, etc.), expense per unit, supplies per unit, revenue per unit, revenue per square foot, and EBITDA		
	g. annual budget and associated performance		
	h. goals/objectives and key strategies		
	i. human resources-related factors, such as turnover rates, productivity, absenteeism, and employee satisfaction		

Appendix F
About the Medical Fitness Association

Mission Statement

The Medical Fitness Association (MFA) is a member-driven, nonprofit organization. Its mission is to foster opportunities for the development and operational success of medically integrated fitness centers. MFA provides industry standards, educational programs, benchmarks, outcome measurements, professional development and networking opportunities for the medical fitness industry.

Vision Statement

To lead a global network of medically integrated fitness centers, programs and professionals in the pursuit of well-being

Code of Ethics

As leaders in the field of medical fitness, MFA professionals pledge:

- To uphold the ethics and mission of the medical fitness profession.
- To set the standard of excellence in the operation of fitness and wellness programs, facilities, and services.
- To operate their programs, services and facilities in a fair, honest, and ethical manner.
- To treat all clients/patients as their employer.
- To ensure that all programs and information delivered to clients are safe, effective, and based on up-to-date research.
- To develop and implement programs and services that improve the quality of life and health of the population they are committed to serve.
- To share "best-of-practice" strategies with the medical-fitness industry at-large.
- To avoid the exploitation of professional relationships for personal gain.

Defining the Future

Medical Fitness Centers are defining the future of professionally administered health and fitness services to an aging population, and are committed to improving outcomes for patients with chronic diseases and multiple risk factors. MFA centers have proven that they can provide a continuum of care, fulfill the mission of their sponsoring institution, and be financially viable in a variety of community settings. As pioneers in the medical fitness industry, MFA professionals believe the future of medically integrated fitness centers is in improving the health status of the communities they serve. In that regard, preventing, rather than treating, illness and disease, is the key to the future of responsible healthcare.

Notable growth and success throughout the medical fitness industry are becoming more prevalent each year. Based on information obtained through industry surveys and other sources, the compound annual growth rate in the number of centers since 1985 is approximately 11.5% beginning with 79 centers. The number of members served has grown to over three million and is projected to reach over four million by 2010.

The Medical Fitness Association, a non-profit organization, founded in 1991, assists medical fitness centers in achieving their full potential. The Association is a professional membership organization whose mission is to ascertain and respond to the needs of medically integrated centers throughout the world. As a resource to the medical fitness industry, MFA is 100% committed to excellence in medical fitness, and is the first association to focus on hospital fitness and wellness.

Benefits of MFA Membership

• *Access to benchmarks for success*
MFA provides members with access to in-depth research on the latest industry trends. MFA report on programs, practices, operations and more. What works? What doesn't? By sharing vital data, MFA helps members formulate standards and protocols that foster excellence and optimize success.

• *Opportunities for professional development*
MFA-sponsored conferences, seminars and educational programs provide exceptional learning and networking opportunities. The goal? Expand the knowledge base of everyone involved—hospital executives, physicians, and medical fitness center professionals alike—and help MFA members improve the overall health of the communities they serve.

• *Recognition as a difference-maker*
As a medically integrated health and fitness center, the programs and services an MFA-affiliated facility offers its community are exceptional and unique. As such, active membership in MFA helps identify a MFA facility or organization as a leader in proactive healthcare.

- *Enhanced public awareness*

MFA has made enhancing public awareness of the benefits of medical fitness a top priority. By cultivating media relationships, providing source material for articles, features and news stories, and distributing press releases, MFA is delivering the message of how essential it is to prevent, rather than treat, disease and illness—a healthcare message that is designed to resonate loudly and clearly with the public.

- *Professional excellence*

The Medical Fitness Association informs, promotes, provides exceptional networking and educational opportunities, serves as an effective advocate, and defines industry-wide standards of professional excellence.

To join MFA, visit www.medicalfitness.org or call 804-897-5701.

For questions regarding standards and guidelines for Medical Fitness Centers and MFA's facility certification program, contact MFA at the following address: P.O. Box 73103, Richmond, VA 23235.

Index